W9-CAV-740

THE DIABETES FOOD & NUTRITION

BIBLE

A Complete Guide to Planning, Shopping, Cooking, and Eating

Hope S. Warshaw, MMSc, RD, CDE, and Robyn Webb, MS

with Foreword by Graham Kerr

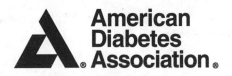

American Diabetes Association

Director, Book Publishing, John Fedor; *Associate Director, Consumer Book Acquisitions,* Sherrye Landrum; *Editor,* Marie McCarren; *Production Manager,* Peggy M. Rote; *Composition,* Circle Graphics, Inc.; *Cover Design,* KSA-Plus Communications; *Nutrient Analysis,* Nutritional Computing Concepts; *Printer,* Port City Press, Inc.

© 2001 by Hope S. Warshaw and Robyn A. Webb. All Rights Reserved. No part of this publication may be reproduced or transmitted in any form or by any means, electronic or mechanical, including duplication, recording, or any information storage and retrieval system, without the prior written permission of the authors.

Printed in the United States of America
1 3 5 7 9 10 8 6 4 2

The suggestions and information contained in this publication are generally consistent with the *Clinical Practice Recommendations* and other policies of the American Diabetes Association, but they do not represent the policy or position of the Association or any of its boards or committees. Reasonable steps have been taken to ensure the accuracy of the information presented. However, the American Diabetes Association cannot ensure the safety or efficacy of any product or service described in this publication. Individuals are advised to consult a physician or other appropriate health care professional before undertaking any diet or exercise program or taking any medication referred to in this publication. Professionals must use and apply their own professional judgment, experience, and training and should not rely solely on the information contained in this publication before prescribing any diet, exercise, or medication. The American Diabetes Association—its officers, directors, employees, volunteers, and members—assumes no responsibility or liability for personal or other injury, loss, or damage that may result from the suggestions or information in this publication.

⊚ The paper in this publication meets the requirements of the ANSI Standard Z39.48-1992 (permanence of paper).

ADA titles may be purchased for business or promotional use or for special sales. For information, please write to Lee Romano Sequeira, Special Sales & Promotions, at the address below.

American Diabetes Association
1701 North Beauregard Street
Alexandria, VA 22311

Library of Congress Cataloging-in-Publication Data

Warshaw, Hope S., 1954–
    The diabetes food and nutrition bible / Hope S. Warshaw, Robyn A. Webb.
    p. cm.
Includes index.
ISBN 1-58040-037-X (pbk. : alk. paper)
    1. Diabetes—Diet therapy. 2. Diabetics—Nutrition. I. Title: Diabetes food and
        nutrition bible. II. Webb, Robyn. III. Title.
RC662 .W314 2001
616.4'620654—dc21   2001022343

Contents

Foreword   v

Introduction   ix

1 **Nutrients: The Big Three** _____   1

2 **Vitamins and Minerals** _____   7

3 **Meal Planning Approaches** _____   15

   Exchange Lists for Meal Planning, 16

   Carbohydrate Counting, 18

   Counting Methods, 19

   The Diabetes Food Pyramid, 20

4 **Grains, Beans, and Starchy Vegetables** _____   23

   Grains, 26

   Beans, Peas, and Lentils, 53

   Starchy Vegetables, 70

   FOCUS ON   Portion Control, 87

5 **Vegetables** _____   91

   FOCUS ON   Water, 120

6 **Fruits** _____   121

   FOCUS ON   Fiber, 153

   FOCUS ON   Fats, 159

7 **Milk and Yogurt** _____ **165**

FOCUS ON   Blood Pressure, 177

8 **Meat and Meat Substitutes** _____ **181**

9 **Fats and Lower-fat Recipes** _____ **235**

10 **Sugars, Sweets, and Sweeteners** _____ **259**

FOCUS ON   Alcohol, 273

11 **Two Weeks of Menus** _____ **277**

FOCUS ON   Finding a Dietitian, 295

12 **The Food Label** _____ **297**

13 **Setting Goals** _____ **311**

FOREWORD

I expect that you share one of my early childhood joys (and challenges): the jigsaw puzzle. First, I would try to group colors that looked alike and then twist and turn pieces to help them fit. With a little help from a friendly adult, I'd start again with the straight edges and corners. Then back to my clusters of sky or sea, continuing the now less-frustrating twist-and-turn assembly.

It's been like that with "our" diabetes, which surfaced after my wife, Treena, had a stroke and heart attack in 1987. Yes, it's my wife, Treena's, disease, but I've loved her ever since I was 11, and if she ever has a challenge, then so do I!

Our earliest attempts to understand her type 2 diabetes were very much like working a jigsaw puzzle—without a picture. We got some fairly blunt advice that, no matter how well meant, really wasn't workable, at least to us. We didn't have a clue about the big picture, only the threat of big trouble if we failed to comply. We sat in our familiar lifestyle, looking at completely unfamiliar demands that, frankly, sounded awful!

So, we fussed and twisted the pieces of advice and got nowhere fast. The sugars rose, the medications increased, we switched to insulin, the weight increased, the emotions roller-coastered, feet hurt, blood pressure was hard to control . . . . We were not happy campers in our new diabetic lifestyle.

We switched educators and found Kitty Carmichael, a perfectly wonderful woman with a passionate desire to see her patients win because they had a real ownership of their disease. Kitty said, "You've got diabetes Treena. I don't, so you deal with it—I can't." It woke us up.

Kitty led us to the straight edges, and Treena and I are filling in the rest of the picture by educating ourselves.

You'll be shown the edges and right angles in this wonderful book by Hope and Robyn. You'll learn how food affects your blood glucose levels and how to move towards a healthier way of eating. You'll see that with a little creativity, you can live well within what can be quite comforting, good-tasting limits.

With the help of experts like Kitty, Hope, and Robyn, we've almost completed the picture. I say almost because science is a moving target. The search for any absolute truth (short of religious faith) is ongoing, so we will never give up wanting more revelation to secure the best possible management of Treena's disease.

If you've bought this book because you have diabetes, then may I suggest you find a creative way to have your partner read it too? If, by chance, you are like me and your loved one has diabetes, then by all means possible, have him or her read this carefully and accept full responsibility. No matter how hard you try to solve their problem, you can't. Only the person with diabetes can negotiate and maintain the creative changes necessary.

I wish you well, whichever role and reason you have before you. You've made an excellent choice of information. Now read, learn, and inwardly digest a very reasonable approach, based upon excellent, up-to-the-minute science.

Treena and I join in prayer for you in your present need. May you experience all the love necessary to live a long life with satisfaction in having done your very best.

Graham Kerr

To people with diabetes:
May the information and advice in
the pages ahead help make the challenge
of eating healthy with diabetes just a bit easier.
— **H.S.W.**

To my husband Allan, for all you do!
— **R.A.W.**

Introduction

When you were diagnosed with diabetes, were you simply given a prescription for a diabetes medication and told to avoid sweets? Were you told to lose weight without any guidance on how? Were you given a preprinted meal plan for a certain number of calories and expected to follow it day in, day out, no questions asked?

Did you sense you were missing important information?

You're about to fill those gaps.

In the following pages, you'll find out how different types of foods affect your blood glucose levels. You'll be able to use that knowledge to help you reach your blood glucose goals. Keeping your blood glucose nearer to normal keeps you feeling your best today and lowers your risk of developing diabetes complications in the future.

Meal planning is the simple act of deciding what to eat. You'll learn about the three most commonly used meal planning systems. These give you a way to make food choices and plan meals without turning your lifestyle upside down.

You'll also learn how to improve your overall health by making healthy food choices. This lowers your risk for heart disease, stroke, and some cancers. Get your family to join you, and they'll lower their risk of developing type 2 diabetes as well.

What will give you all these rewards? Some kind of restrictive, boring "diet"? Absolutely not! You may be surprised to learn that there are no longer any "forbidden" foods or special "diabetic diets."

Healthy eating is healthy eating. But it's different from the way many Americans eat. Ideally, to meet the challenge, you'll work with a dietitian who specializes in diabetes. He or she will help you decide which eating habits you might want to change to achieve your diabetes goals, help you choose a meal planning tool that works best for your needs, and coach and support you on an ongoing basis. Learn how to find a dietitian on page 295.

But there is much you can learn on your own. Whether you're ready for just a few changes or a major overhaul, this book will guide you, with:

- Hundreds of tips on easy ways to work healthy food choices into your meals.

- Nutrition Superstars. These foods, from avocado to leafy green vegetables to wheat germ, are nutrition powerhouses. One may be a good source of fiber and certain vitamins, another may be an excellent source of calcium. Whatever their assets, these foods give you an above-average dose of nutrition for your calories. They're what nutrition experts call "nutritionally dense foods." You'll find tips on how to buy, store, and cook with these Nutrition Superstars.

- Over 100 recipes for healthy, flavorful meals, many of which feature a Nutrition Superstar (those are marked with a star). Each recipe has the nutrition information you need for diabetes meal planning whether you use the exchange system, carbohydrate counting, fat and calorie counting, or any other method.

Eat well and enjoy your journey.

Nutrients
The Big Three

Your body gets energy from three main sources:

- carbohydrate
- protein
- fat

Each has a different effect on blood glucose levels.

CARBOHYDRATE

Nearly all of the carbohydrate you eat ends up as glucose in your bloodstream. The two other major sources of energy, protein and fat, have little direct impact on blood glucose levels. Therefore for blood glucose control, you'll want to pay close attention to the total amount of carbohydrate you eat.

Sugars vs. Starches

There are two categories of carbohydrates: sugars and starches.

Sugars include glucose, fructose, and lactose.

Starches are long chains of glucose units hooked together. Grains, pasta, and potatoes contain starch.

When eaten, carbohydrates—whether they are sugars or starches—are, for the most part, broken down into glucose.

Once foods are broken down into glucose, your body doesn't know whether the glucose came from a bowl of pasta, jelly beans, or an oatmeal cookie. To the body, glucose is just its favorite source of energy.

For many years health professionals advised people with diabetes to limit sugars. It seemed to make sense that sugars would be absorbed more quickly into the bloodstream and therefore raise blood glucose more quickly than starches.

Today, from many years of research, we know that the effect on blood glucose is virtually the same whether you eat sugars or starch. It's the total amount of carbohydrate you consume each time you eat, rather than the source, that determines how much glucose reaches your bloodstream.

In fact, fruits (which contain fructose) and milk (which contains lactose) have been shown to have less of an effect on blood glucose levels than some starches. Sucrose (table sugar) has less of an effect on blood glucose than bread, rice, or potatoes.

How Much?

Carbohydrate is your body's main and preferred energy source, whether it's energy to keep your heart beating or energy to walk around the block. Typically, carbohydrate makes up 40% to 60% of calorie intake.

What foods contain carbohydrate? Most people would first name bread, cereal, rice, and pasta. All these foods are starches, and most of their calories come from carbohydrate, along with a few calories from protein.

Many other foods contain carbohydrate. A few may surprise you. They're covered in various chapters of this book.

Foods With Carbohydrate	Chapter
Breads, cereals, and grains	Starches
Starchy vegetables (corn, potatoes)	Starches
Beans, peas, and lentils	Starches
Crackers and snacks	Starches
Fruit and fruit juice	Fruit
Milk, yogurt	Milk
Sugary foods (gum drops, regular soda, fruit drinks)	Sugars and Sweets
Sweets (cakes, cookies, pies, candy)	Sugars and Sweets

When you're estimating the effect a meal will have on your blood glucose level, you'll consider all sources of carbohydrate—starches, fruits, vegetables, dairy foods, and sweets.

Insulin Steps In

Carbohydrate gets broken down into glucose, and the glucose moves into the bloodstream. There's one more step before the body can use glucose for energy: getting the glucose into cells. For that final step, you need two things: insulin, and cells that respond to insulin.

If you have type 1 diabetes, your pancreas doesn't make any insulin. You use injected insulin to move glucose into cells.

If you have type 2 diabetes, you likely have some degree of what's called insulin resistance. Your cells don't respond well to insulin. You can help your body use insulin better by:

- Becoming more active.
- Losing a modest amount (10 to 20 pounds) of excess weight (if you are overweight).

Your health care provider might also prescribe oral diabetes medication. Many people with type 2 take one or more pills. About 30% to 40% of people with type 2 diabetes require insulin injections, especially after they have had diabetes for a number of years.

Fiber

Fiber is carbohydrate, but you can't digest it, so it doesn't raise blood glucose levels.

Fiber has numerous health benefits. A healthy intake of fiber is 20 to 35 grams a day from a variety of foods. Most Americans get only 11 to 13 grams a day. If you eat more servings of whole grains, legumes, fruits, and vegetables, you'll increase your fiber intake. See Focus on Fiber, p. 153.

PROTEIN

Your body needs many different proteins to function properly. Proteins repair tissue. During phases of growth, such as infancy and pregnancy, proteins help form new body tissues. Enzymes, antibodies, and hormones are proteins. In fact, the hormone insulin is a protein.

Proteins are made up of 20 different amino acids. These building blocks of proteins come from the protein-containing foods you eat.

The body can't make what are called essential amino acids, so you must get them from the protein-containing foods you eat. There is a larger group of non-essential amino acids. The body is able to make all the non-essential amino acids as long as you eat sufficient essential amino acids and enough carbohydrate and fat.

You might be familiar with the terms "complete protein" and "incomplete protein." A complete protein is a food that contains all nine essential amino acids. Examples of complete proteins are meat, poultry, seafood, dairy foods, eggs, and soy products. Incomplete proteins are missing one or more essential amino acids. Beans and peas, grains, nuts, seeds, and vegetables contain incomplete protein.

Years ago it was thought that to be healthy you had to consume all the nine essential amino acids at each meal. That meant you had to either eat an animal product, or mix and match grains, beans, and seeds to get the full complement of essential amino acids at each meal. Today, nutrition experts believe that if you eat a variety of incomplete proteins during the day and enough calories, the body can make all the necessary proteins. This is a particularly important topic for vegetarians, who may choose to eat few, if any, complete proteins.

Protein and Blood Glucose

For many years, it was thought that about half the protein in a meal was converted into glucose, and that this happened slowly. Therefore, it was thought that protein raised blood glucose more slowly than carbohydrate.

After more research, these theories are now in question. It is now known that protein stimulates the production of insulin in people with type 2 diabetes. This small rise in insulin does lower blood glucose.

In people with type 1 diabetes taking enough insulin, protein has little effect on blood glucose. However larger intakes of protein can increase blood glucose and lead to the need for an increase in insulin.

The advice about protein today is to monitor your blood glucose and see what works best for you. Some people feel they do better with some protein at each meal and snack, yet for others it doesn't make a difference. In reality, with the small amount of protein you should eat, it's difficult to spread such a small quantity across so many meals and snacks. Also, protein often adds unwanted calories from the fat that comes with it.

How Much?

The recommended dietary allowance (RDA) for protein for nonpregnant adults is 0.8 grams per kilogram of body weight or about 0.4 grams per pound. That's about 50 grams of protein for a 120-pound woman and about 70 grams of protein for a 170-pound man.

At the RDA, protein would make up about 10% of total daily calories. Americans eat about 14% to 18% of calories as protein.

Simply from a health standpoint, eating a protein intake nearer the RDA and with a greater number of choices from the non-animal protein group is beneficial in several ways. It helps you eat less total fat, saturated fat, and cholesterol. Second, it saves room on your plate for grains, fruits, and vegetables—the foods that are loaded with fiber, vitamins, and minerals.

If you have diabetic kidney disease, you may be advised to eat less excess protein and get down to the RDA.

Where's the Protein?

When you think of protein, do you think first of red meat, poultry, and seafood? Foods from several other food groups provide protein as well.

Foods That Contain Protein	Chapter
Red meat, poultry, seafood	Meat
Cheese	Meat
Eggs	Meat
Soy products	Meat
Peanut butter	Meat, Fat
Beans, peas, and lentils	Starches
Milk, yogurt	Milk
Starches	Starches
Vegetables	Vegetables
Nuts	Fats

FAT

With all the negative talk about fat, you might wonder whether fat does any good. It does! The body needs a small amount of fat to provide essential fatty acids; carry the fat-soluble vitamins A, D, E, and K; maintain healthy skin; and produce components of some hormones.

Fat in your food has very little effect on your blood glucose levels. But the kinds of fat you eat do affect your blood lipid levels, which affects your risk of heart disease.

We discuss types of fat and fat intake in more detail in Focus on Fat, p. 159, and in the Meat, Milk, and Fat chapters.

Vitamins and Minerals

Vitamins are essential to the proper functioning of the body. They must be eaten in sufficient quantities to maintain health.

For the past two decades, the Recommended Dietary Allowances (RDAs), published by the Food and Nutrition Board of the National Academy of Sciences (NAS), have been the last word in defining an adequate nutrition intake. The RDAs are defined as the levels of intake of essential nutrients that, on the basis of scientific knowledge, are judged to be adequate to meet the known nutrient needs of nearly all healthy people.

The RDAs have been updated many times since 1941. In recent years, the knowledge about the impact of nutrients on health and the prevention of disease has expanded dramatically. To help people integrate new and future science into sensible guidelines, several new categories of recommendations are being developed by NAS under the heading of Dietary Reference Intakes (DRIs). The DRI term refers to four reference values to be applied to all nutrients.

■ *Recommended Dietary Allowance (RDA)*: The average daily nutrient intake that is sufficient to meet the nutrition needs of nearly all healthy individuals in an age group or life stage.

■ *Adequate Intake (AI)*: A recommended daily intake level based on observed or experimentally determined approximations of nutrient intake by a group (or groups) of healthy people. AI is used when there is insufficient science to determine an RDA.

■ *Estimated Average Requirement (EAR)*: A nutrient intake value that is estimated to meet the requirement of half the healthy people in an age or life-stage group. It is used to assess adequacy of intakes of population groups and to develop RDAs.

■ *Tolerable Upper Intake Level (UL)*: The highest level of daily nutrient intake that is likely to pose no risk of adverse health effects to almost all people in the general population. As nutrient intakes increase above the UL, the risk of adverse effects increases.

At present, the FDA continues to use a set of recommendations called Reference Daily Intakes or RDIs for 19 vitamins and minerals as guidelines for food labeling and nutrition claims. On food labels, the RDIs are also referred to as Daily Values or DVs.

Once the NAS has set all the DRIs, FDA will review the findings of the Food and Nutrition Board of the National Academy of Sciences and revise the nutrient guidelines used in food labeling as needed. This is not predicted to happen until the mid- to late-2000s.

From Food or Pills?

The American Diabetes Association's position is that as long as your diet is good, you probably don't need vitamin pills. However, people on weight-reducing diets, strict vegetarians, woman who are pregnant or breastfeeding, people taking medications known to alter vitamin and mineral status, people whose blood glucose levels are consistently high, or people in the hospital for long periods of time may need vitamin or mineral supplements.

Nutrients that the body needs in only very small amounts—called micronutrients—are still being identified. A vitamin pill doesn't take the place of choosing to eat a variety of healthy foods including plenty of fruits, vegetables, enriched or unprocessed grains, and legumes.

WATER-SOLUBLE VITAMINS

Water-soluble vitamins (vitamin C and the B vitamins) are carried in the bloodstream. The body uses the amount it needs and then gets rid of the extra in the urine. They aren't stored, so you need to consume water-soluble vitamins regularly to stay healthy.

Water-soluble vitamins can be destroyed more easily than fat-soluble vitamins in food preparation, cooking, and storing.

Vitamin B1: Thiamin

Thiamin is involved in many steps of the process of converting carbohydrate into a usable form of energy—glucose. The hull, or outer layer, of grains is high in thiamin. Since 1942, the Enrichment Act requires that thiamin be added to flour and cereals to compensate for the loss of thiamin that occurs when grain is milled and processed.

Good food sources: Whole grains, legumes (beans and peas) and seeds, pork, bread made with enriched white flour, and fortified cereals.

Vitamin B2: Riboflavin

Riboflavin is needed to release the body's stored energy for use and is involved in many steps in the breakdown of carbohydrate, protein, and fat. It is involved with the functioning of vitamins B6 and niacin. Ultraviolet light, such as sunlight, destroys riboflavin, which is the reason milk is sold in plastic containers that are opaque or waxed paper containers.

> *Good food sources:* Dairy products, eggs, liver, some seafood, whole grains, fortified cereals, baked goods made with enriched flour, and some green vegetables—asparagus, broccoli, and spinach.

Vitamin B3: Niacin

Niacin is involved in many steps in the breakdown of carbohydrate, protein, and fat. It is also important in the health of skin, and the digestive and nervous systems.

> *Good food sources:* Foods rich in protein, such as fish, meat, poultry, and peanut butter; breads made with enriched flour; and fortified cereals.

Vitamin B5: Pantothenic Acid

Pantothenic acid is involved in the breakdown of carbohydrate, protein, and fat. It plays a role in making fatty acids, cholesterol, and some hormones. Milling destroys a lot of pantothenic acid in grains.

> *Good food sources:* Whole grains, legumes, fish, meat, poultry, and some fruits and vegetables.

Vitamin B6: Pyridoxine

Pyridoxine is involved in the breakdown of protein and building non-essential proteins in the body. It is necessary to produce red blood cells and in the proper functioning of nerve tissue. Processing of foods, heating, and exposure to ultraviolet light reduces the content of pyridoxine in foods.

> *Good food sources:* Chicken, fish, pork, whole grains, legumes.

Folate/Folic Acid

Folate is the form of the vitamin found in foods; folic acid is the synthetic form used in supplements and fortified foods.

Folic acid is essential for the creation of new cells (DNA and RNA). It is important in the formation of hemoglobin in red blood cells, and during pregnancy for the growth of the fetus. It has been determined that pregnant women who don't consume enough folate, especially in the early stages of pregnancy, increase their risk of having a baby with neural tube defects (spina bifida). Therefore, as of 1998 the FDA requires that all grain products (breads, cereals, and pasta) be fortified with 140 mcg folic acid per kilogram of grain with the goal of increasing the folic acid intake of Americans.

Good food sources: Leafy green vegetables are the richest source by far. Legumes, oranges, whole grains, wheat germ, and fortified foods noted above.

Vitamin B12: Cobalamin

Vitamin B12, which is the more commonly used name, is needed along with folic acid to make red blood cells. Vitamin B12 is involved in building and maintaining the covering that protects nerve fibers. A deficiency of B12 can cause a form of anemia, called pernicious anemia. B12 is fairly stable in foods.

Nearly a third of people over 50 years old can no longer produce enough "intrinsic factor"—a substance in the stomach lining—to adequately absorb B12. They need to get B12 from a supplement or from cereal that is fortified with B12.

Good food sources: Found exclusively in foods of animal origin—meats, dairy products, and eggs. It is not found in plant foods, and sufficient intake may be a problem for strict vegetarians.

Vitamin C

Vitamin C is important in forming the protein collagen, which is part of the body's connective tissue. Collagen helps heal cuts and wounds and keeps you from bruising by maintaining firm blood vessels. Vitamin C protects you from infection by keeping the immune system healthy. It also increases the absorption of iron from foods of plant sources (the non-heme form of iron). People who smoke have an increased need for vitamin C.

Good food sources: Citrus fruits, oranges, and grapefruits. Broccoli, green pepper, and strawberries.

Biotin

Biotin is important in the breakdown of carbohydrate, protein, and fat. Biotin is produced by the natural bacteria in the intestine, so getting enough biotin is rarely a problem.

Good food sources: Egg yolk, liver, yeast, and cereals.

FAT-SOLUBLE VITAMINS

Fat-soluble vitamins are carried in the bloodstream attached to fats. The body stores fat-soluble vitamins, so you don't need regular amounts as much as you do with water-soluble vitamins.

Vitamin A

Vitamin A is best known for its role in eyesight. But it is also important for healthy skin, and the mucous membranes of the body—mouth, lungs, intestines. It plays a role in the body's immunity, growth of bones, production of red blood cells, and the lining of nerve cells. In the form of carotenoids, which are mainly found in fruits and vegetables, vitamin A is an antioxidant. Beta carotene is one of the more familiar antioxidants, or carotenoids that convert to vitamin A.

> *Good food sources:* Two categories of sources: 1) in the form of retinol from foods of animal origin—liver, eggs, milk fortified with vitamin A; 2) in the form of carotenoids that convert to vitamin A in the body—orange, red, yellow, and dark-green leafy vegetables.

Vitamin D

Vitamin D is essential for increasing the absorption of calcium into the body. It also regulates the breakdown of calcium and phosphorus and promotes the growth of strong bones. Most of the intake of vitamin D is not from food, it's from the action of sunlight (ultraviolet light), which forms vitamin D in the skin. With enough sunlight, there is no need for vitamin D.

The NAS report in 1997 indicated a higher need for vitamin D than previously given because people are not being exposed to as much sunlight today, and many people use sunscreen when they are in the sunlight. An even higher need is recommended for older adults because they might not be as efficiently converting vitamin D from sunshine. They should either take a multivitamin that provides enough vitamin D or take a calcium supplement that is fortified with vitamin D.

> *Good food sources:* Fortified milk, egg yolks, butter, liver.

Vitamin E

Vitamin E acts as an antioxidant to prevent damage to cells, which may reduce the risk of some cancers, and heart disease. There are several forms of vitamin E. These are various forms of tocopherols. The most active is alpha-tocopherol. According to the American Diabetes Association, studies show that vitamin E levels are variable in people with diabetes. There are thus far no studies that confirm that vitamin E supplementation has any benefit in people with diabetes. It is noted that more studies are required before any recommendation for supplementation is made.

Good food sources: Foods that are high in unsaturated fats—vegetable oils, margarine, and salad dressing; nuts, seeds, and wheat germ; unprocessed grains.

Vitamin K

Vitamin K is important for normal blood clotting and to create proteins. Vitamin K can be obtained from nonfood sources—bacteria in the gastrointestinal tract make vitamin K.

Good food sources: Green leafy vegetables—spinach, broccoli, kale, greens; cabbage, egg, and milk.

MINERALS

Minerals are found in soil and from there get into our food supply. The amount of various minerals found in foods depends on the mineral content in which the foods are grown. Quite a bit of variation exists.

Calcium

Calcium is the most abundant mineral in the body. However, it is the mineral that many Americans don't get enough of. Most of the calcium is in the bones, although there is a constant flow of calcium between the bones and the bloodstream. Calcium is also involved in the transmission of nerve impulses, blood clotting, muscle contraction, and absorption of vitamin B12. Calcium is regulated by hormones and requires a hormone made with vitamin D for this process. Vitamin D is needed for the proper absorption of calcium, so an insufficient amount of vitamin D will decrease the amount of calcium absorbed.

Good food sources: Milk (look for calcium-fortified fat-free milk to get your biggest bang of calcium), yogurt, cheese, and other dairy foods are your best sources. Dark-green leafy vegetables and legumes are also good sources.

Iron

Iron is a necessary component of hemoglobin. Hemoglobin carries oxygen in the blood throughout the body. Vitamin C helps increase the absorption of the type of iron found in fruits and vegetables.

If you take both a calcium and iron supplement, take them at different times of the day to get better absorption of each mineral.

Good food sources: Lean meat, fish and poultry, organ meats, legumes, nuts and seeds, whole grains, and green leafy vegetables.

Phosphorus

Phosphorus is another abundant mineral in the body and most of it is in the bones and teeth. Phosphorus is involved in bone formation; in getting energy out of the foods you eat; regulating the breakdown of carbohydrates, proteins, and fats; and is part of DNA and RNA.

Good food sources: Foods high in protein—eggs, fish, meat, poultry; milk and dairy products; legumes and nuts.

Iodine

Iodine is part of thyroid hormones. Thyroid hormones play many roles in the body including regulation of metabolic rate, body temperature, and muscle and nerve function. At one time the development of a goiter, an enlarged thyroid gland, was a common sign of iodine deficiency. To solve this problem iodine was, and continues to be, added to a common ingredient—salt.

Good food sources: Near the seashore, seafood, water, and the mist from the ocean are sources. Inland the amount of iodine in foods depends on many factors. The most reliable source of iodine is iodized salt. When you purchase salt, make sure it is iodized salt.

Magnesium

Magnesium helps relax muscles and helps conduct nerve impulses. It activates many of the body's enzymes to complete its chemical reactions. More than half the body's magnesium is in the bones.

More than 80% of the magnesium is lost from whole grains when they are milled, and magnesium is not added back when flour is enriched. According to the American Diabetes Association, there may be a need for magnesium supplementation in people whose blood glucose levels are consistently high, or who are on a category of high blood pressure medications called diuretics.

Good food sources: Legumes, nuts and seeds, unprocessed whole grains, dark-green leafy vegetables, and bananas.

Zinc

Zinc is necessary for the breakdown of protein, carbohydrates, fats, and alcohol. Zinc is needed to make proteins, DNA and RNA, and insulin. It helps heal wounds and helps us taste foods. Zinc is involved in growth and development, so it's important for children and pregnant women.

Good food sources: Seafood, meat, wheat germ, and tofu.

Selenium

Selenium is part of an enzyme that functions in the body as an antioxidant. Selenium also works closely with vitamin E, another antioxidant. It is known that selenium supplements can be dangerous.

Good food sources: Seafood, meats, and organ meats. Whole grains and seeds contain selenium, but the amount depends on the selenium content of the soil they were grown in.

Copper

Copper is involved with making red blood cells, absorbing and transferring iron, healing wounds, forming bone, and making collagen.

Good food sources: Legumes, organ meat, nuts and seeds.

Fluoride

Fluoride is best known for its role in hardening tooth enamel. It thus helps protect teeth from decay. Fluoride also helps strengthen bones.

Good sources: Fluoride is not widely distributed in foods. The main source of fluoride is fluoridated water. In areas where the natural fluoride in the water is low, the area may fluoridate the water to a level recommended by the American Dental Association. In addition, fluoride might be prescribed to infants, and dentists may prescribe fluoride treatments at various life stages.

Chromium

Chromium helps the body break down carbohydrates and fats. Chromium works with insulin to help the cells get glucose inside to be able to release energy. Research has shown that people with a chromium deficiency may have difficulty controlling their blood glucose levels; however, according to the American Diabetes Association, it is unlikely that most people with diabetes are chromium deficient. Several studies conducted in people with diabetes who were not chromium deficient have not shown any improvement in blood glucose with chromium supplementation.

Good food sources: Meat, organ meats, whole grains, and cheese.

SECTION 3

Meal Planning Approaches

Right off the bat, let's dispel a few myths about diabetes meal planning.

Myth *The only approach for diabetes meal planning is the Exchange System.*

Fact The Exchange System, formally called Exchange Lists for Meal Planning, is just one way to plan meals if you have diabetes.

Myth *A preprinted meal plan for a certain number of calories is all the information and advice you need to eat right to control your diabetes.*

Fact This has never been true! Over the years millions of preprinted meal plans have, unfortunately, been distributed to people with diabetes. But educators have learned that people don't change their food choices or eating behaviors easily or just because they have been diagnosed with diabetes.

Myth *Once you choose a meal planning approach, that will be the one you use forever.*

Fact The meal planning approach you use can change as your diabetes, diabetes goals, and motivation changes. For example, you might start off using a meal planning method that is easy for you to understand. Then a few years later, you decide you want to more closely control your blood glucose levels. Together with an educator, you can explore a more structured method.

KEEPING CARBOHYDRATE THE "SAME"
Many meal plans for people with diabetes are designed to encourage you to eat similar amounts of carbohydrate at similar times each day. That means that every day, your breakfast contains about the same amount of carbohydrate. Likewise, your lunches and dinners will contain about the same amount of carbohydrate.

15

Work with a diabetes educator to help you select a meal planning approach and develop a meal plan just for you. An educator can also help you solve the problems of everyday food issues with diabetes. Challenges will always come up, whether it's a special event, travel, or the flu.

If one system doesn't work, try another. Feel free to say, "I don't understand this system," or "It just doesn't work for me," or "OK, I'm ready to read food labels more and weigh and measure my foods more consistently when I eat at home."

Ready? Explore!

Exchange Lists for Meal Planning a.k.a. The Exchange System

To begin, a bit of history. You may have the impression that the Exchange System is *the* way people with diabetes learn to plan meals. That statement was truer years ago than it is today.

The exchange system started back in 1950 when the American Diabetes Association, The American Dietetic Association, and the United States Public Health Service developed the Exchange Lists for Meal Planning. The goal was to make meal planning easier for people with diabetes and to develop a consistent approach so health professionals could have a common language. Since 1950, the exchange system has been revised a number of times. The last revision was in 1995.

Though other meal planning approaches—some more general and some more structured—have gotten popular, the exchange system is still a viable meal planning approach. If it works for you, great! If not, perhaps it's time to try another approach.

How It Works

The exchange system categorizes foods into three main groups:

Carbohydrate. Foods in the carbohydrate group are divided into five food groups: starch, fruit, milk, other carbohydrates (sugary foods and sweets), and vegetables. The user can swap foods between the starch, fruit, milk, and "other carbohydrate" groups, because foods in these groups contain about the same amount of carbohydrate per serving—12 to 15 grams. Foods in the vegetable group contain less carbohydrate.

Meat and meat substitutes (eggs, cheese, soy). The meat group is divided into four lists: very lean meats, lean meats, medium-fat meats, and high-fat meats.

Fat. The fat group is divided into monounsaturated, polyunsaturated, and saturated fats.

Groups/Lists	Carbohydrate (g)	Protein (g)	Fat (g)	Calories
Carbohydrate Group				
Starch	15	3	1 or less	80
Fruit	15	---	---	60
Milk				
Fat-free	12	8	0–3	90
Low-fat	12	8	5	120
Whole	12	8	8	150
Other carbohydrates	15	varies	varies	varies
Vegetables	5	2	---	25
Meat and Meat Substitute Group				
Very Lean	---	7	0–1	35
Lean	---	7	3	55
Medium-fat	---	7	5	75
High-fat	---	7	8	100
Fat Group	---	---	5	45

An exchange system meal plan doesn't dictate exactly what foods you will eat. Instead, you choose from the "exchange lists": lists of foods (with amounts) with similar nutritional make-up. For example, here are three foods from the starch group: one slice of bread, a small baked potato, 3/4 cup of unsweetened dry cereal. Each of these has about the same amount of carbohydrate, protein, and fat.

A clear advantage of choosing the exchange system is that it's still the common language when communicating about food and diabetes. Cookbooks, magazine articles about food, and even some food labels use the exchange system.

Exchanges Lists for Meal Planning, American Diabetes Association, Inc.,
The American Dietetic Association, 1995.

Official Pocket Guide to Diabetic Exchanges, American Diabetes Association, Inc.,
The American Dietetic Association, 1997.

Carbohydrate Counting

Within one to two hours of eating, 90% to 100% of the digestible starches and sugars turn up in your blood as glucose. So the amount of carbohydrate you eat determines the amount of medication you need to cover the rise in blood glucose from meals and snacks. That's the basis for "carb counting."

There are two ways to count carbs:

Grams of carbohydrate.

Carbohydrate choices. A carbohydrate choice has 15 grams of carbohydrate.

There are two approaches to carb counting:

Basic Carb Counting. You and your dietitian or diabetes educator work out the number of carbohydrate choices or grams for you to eat at each meal and snack. In this way, you keep your carbohydrate intake consistent.

Basic carbohydrate counting can be appropriate for anyone with diabetes.

Advanced Carb Counting. With advanced carb counting, you identify the number of carbohydrate grams or choices in a meal or snack by reading labels, referencing carbohydrate counting resources, and weighing and measuring portions. Then you take the amount of insulin needed to cover that amount of carbohydrate. To do this, you apply your individualized carbohydrate-to-insulin ratio (grams of carbohydrate to units of insulin) that you and your diabetes educator have worked out. The rapid- or short-acting insulin you take before meals is adjusted.

This method is appropriate for people who take insulin at each meal or who use an insulin pump. To some extent, it can also be used by people who take the oral medication repaglinide (Prandin) or nateglinide (Starlix).

Advanced carbohydrate counting is a popular meal planning method, because it allows more flexibility in a meal plan.

FOR MORE HELP

The Diabetes Carbohydrate and Fat Gram Guide, 2nd ed., Holzmeister, American Diabetes Association, Inc., 2000.

ADA Guide to Healthy Restaurant Eating, Warshaw, American Diabetes Association, Inc., 1998.

ADA Complete Guide to Carb Counting, Warshaw and Kulkarni, American Diabetes Association, Inc., 2001.

Counting Methods

Another approach to meal planning is to count calories and/or grams of fat. These methods are most appropriate if you have type 2 diabetes and are overweight, because weight loss is a major goal.

You and an educator establish a range for the calories and number of fat grams you should eat each day. You learn how to keep precise food records. You look up the calories and/or grams of fat in the foods you choose to eat and record these on your food records.

This meal planning approach is particularly good if you need to become more aware of what you eat as well as to learn the number of calories and grams of fat in foods.

While you can count just calories or grams of fat, it's best to count both. That's because if you just count fat grams, it's easy to get carried away with fat-free and low-fat foods. Often these foods trade their fat calories for carbohydrate calories.

FOR MORE HELP

The Diabetes Carbohydrate and Fat Gram Guide, 2nd ed., Holzmeister, American Diabetes Association, Inc., 2000.

ADA Guide to Healthy Restaurant Eating, Warshaw, American Diabetes Association, Inc., 1998.

ADA Guide to Convenience Food Counts, Holzmeister, American Diabetes Association, Inc., 2001.

The Diabetes Food Pyramid

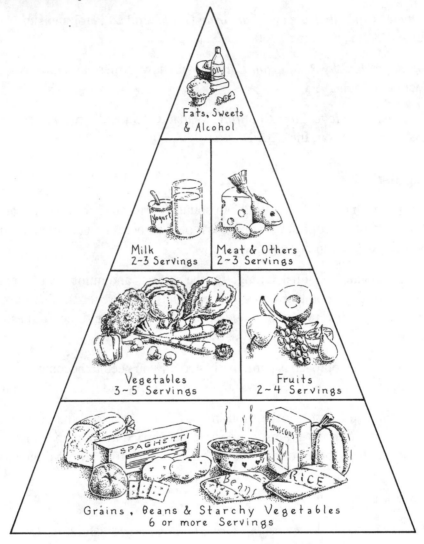

You're probably familiar with the United States Department of Agriculture (USDA) Food Guide Pyramid. It's on many food packages. The shape of the Food Guide Pyramid guides people to a healthy diet. Breads, cereals, rice, and pasta make up the base of the Food Guide Pyramid. That means a healthy diet has more servings of those foods and fewer servings of sweets and fats, which are found in the top, smaller sections the Food Guide Pyramid.

In 1995, the American Diabetes Association and The American Dietetic Association adapted the USDA Food Guide Pyramid for people with diabetes. A few foods were shifted into different categories based on their effect on blood glucose. Potatoes, for example, are higher in carbohydrate than most vegetables. A serving of potatoes will have a greater effect on blood glucose than a serving of green beans. So potatoes and other starchy vegetables were switched from vegetables to the bottom layer of the Diabetes Food Pyramid: Grains, Beans, and Starchy Vegetables.

The Diabetes Food Pyramid serves two roles: It's a diabetes meal planning tool as well as a guide to healthy eating. You and a diabetes educator can design meal plans so you get similar amounts of carbohydrate at meals and snacks while eating according to the pyramid.

The recipes in this book are organized into the six sections of the Diabetes Food Pyramid.

FOR MORE HELP

Diabetes Meal Planning, Made Easy, 2nd ed., Warshaw, American Diabetes Association, Inc., 2000.

Q I've heard of the Glycemic Index. Should I learn to use it in planning my meals?

A The Glycemic Index of foods is a concept that was popularized in the early 1980s. Researchers studied how quickly or slowly various carbohydrate foods raised blood glucose. They then ranked these foods. Glucose was the standard and was given the score of 100.

It had been thought that foods with sugar raised blood glucose very quickly. The glycemic index research showed this wasn't true. It showed that potatoes, for example, raise blood glucose more quickly than does fruit, and legumes raise blood glucose quite slowly.

This information was clearly valuable. However, this method of analyzing foods looks at one food at a time. This isn't how we eat. We eat several foods at a time. Also, many factors affect how quickly foods raise blood glucose, such as the ripeness of the fruit or vegetable, preparation, whether the food is cooked or raw, and how quickly or slowly the person eats. So as a meal planning tool, the Glycemic Index doesn't prove helpful for most people.

However, you may find it helpful to develop your "personal glycemic index." You might find that a certain food simply raises your blood glucose very quickly. But don't jump to conclusions. Try the food several times and make sure your blood glucose isn't rising quickly or too high because the portion is large or because of other foods you ate at the same time.

WHICH IS BEST FOR ME?

The educator you work with should help you choose a meal planning approach that matches your lifestyle, abilities, and needs. Keep in mind that the meal planning approach you choose can and likely will change over the years as you and your diabetes change.

- Do you need a rigid plan to follow? One with limited food choices? Or will a meal planning approach with minimal structure be more appropriate for your needs and personality?

- Do you want a meal planning approach that is very simple to understand?

- Do you need to lose weight to manage your diabetes or has weight control never been a problem for you? If you have attempted a number of weight loss programs, consider what type of plan you have been more or less successful with.

- Are you willing to do calculations before eating each meal to gain a level of flexibility or does that not appeal to you?

- Are you willing to record your food intake for a period of time to observe your food intake and the impact of some changes, or are you simply never going to be willing to complete food records?

- All methods of meal planning require some weighing and measuring of foods for success. However, some methods, carbohydrate counting for one, require a long-term commitment to weighing and measuring foods. Are you willing to do that?

- Are you willing to read food labels? All methods of meal planning require that you read food labels in the supermarket. However, some methods, carbohydrate counting for one, require a long-term commitment to reading food labels.

- Is your life fairly structured—breakfast, lunch, and dinner are at about the same time each day and you take a walk at the same time each day? In addition, do you take no diabetes medicines or at least none that can cause low blood glucose? Or do you never quite know when breakfast, lunch, or dinner will be or when you will get called away for an urgent matter? Have you chosen a medication regimen for its level of flexibility and thus need a meal planning approach that dovetails?

Grains, Beans, and Starchy Vegetables

The Foundation of Healthy Eating

This symbol indicates the Nutrition Superstars. When you include these foods in your meals, you get extra value for your choices.

RECIPES

GRAINS

⚹ Barley and Brown Rice in Many Ways _____ 30

⚹ Nutty Blueberry Pancakes _____ 31

  Couscous Many Ways_____ 32

⚹ Basic Quinoa_____ 33

⚹ Quinoa Stuffed Peppers_____ 34

⚹ Quinoa Salad _____ 35

⚹ Basic Wild Rice _____ 36

⚹ Wild Rice Salad_____ 37

⚹ Italian Wild Rice Pilaf_____ 38

  Confetti Rice and Beans_____ 39

⚹ Basic Polenta _____ 40

  Cranberry Rice_____ 42

Pasta

Fusilli with Sage and Peppers_____ 44

Pasta Primavera _____ 45

Penne Pasta with Basil Vinaigrette _____ 46

Asian Noodle Salad _____ 47

Oven-dried Tomatoes, Garlic, and Pasta ___ 48

Asian Scallop Fettucine _____ 49

Angel Hair with Feta and Capers_____ 50

Chicken, Spinach, and Shell Soup _____ 51

Marinara Sauce_____ 52

Pesto Sauce_____ 52

BEANS, PEAS, AND LENTILS

➤ Almond-Pesto White Beans
with Vegetables _____ 56

➤ Bow Tie Pasta with Sun-dried Tomato Pesto
and White Beans _____ 57

➤ Colorful Lentil Salad _____ 58

➤ Pasta Fagioli _____ 59

➤ Bean Salad in Many Ways _____ 60

➤ Black Bean Jicama Salad _____ 62

➤ Spanish Black Bean Soup _____ 63

➤ White Bean Chili _____ 64

➤ Red Bean Creole _____ 65

➤ Tex-Mex Beans _____ 66

➤ Shrimp and Bean Skillet _____ 67

➤ Herbed Chickpeas and Potatoes _____ 68

➤ Couscous Bean Pilaf _____ 69

STARCHY VEGETABLES

➤ Sweet Potato Fries _____ 71

➤ Festive Sweet Potatoes _____ 72

Foil-Roasted Herb Potatoes _____ 74

Creamy Mashed Potatoes _____ 75

Twice-Baked Potatoes _____ 76

Chive Corn Pudding _____ 79

Vegetable Burritos _____ 80

Glazed Parsnips _____ 81

Butternut Squash and Pear Soup _____ 82

Yes, It's True— starches, as well as other foods with carbohydrate, raise blood glucose. That's why the first inclination of many people with diabetes is to skip and skimp on starches. Don't!

MAKE STARCHES THE STAR

Starches are among the healthiest foods to eat.

■ Unless you add it, starches have almost no fat. Consider a slice of whole-grain bread or a bowl of oatmeal.

■ Starches have a small amount of protein, and it's not animal protein. That means minimal to no saturated fat and no cholesterol.

■ Starches are generally good sources of some B vitamins, such as thiamin (B1), riboflavin (B2), and niacin (B3). They're good sources of the minerals magnesium, copper, and iron. The orange starchy vegetables—winter, acorn, hubbard, and butternut squash; pumpkin; and sweet potatoes and yams—top the chart for carotenoids, most of which convert to vitamin A in the body. Dry cereal and dried peas and beans are excellent sources of folate.

■ Overall, starches are the best sources of dietary fiber in the diet. (See Focus on Fiber, p. 153)

Grains, beans, and starchy vegetables form the foundation of the Diabetes Food Pyramid. The message is to eat more servings of these foods than of any of the other food groups.

Let starches be the centerpiece of the meal instead of only a side dish. We know, this has not been the American way, but make it your way of eating. For example, you might want to have a bowl of whole-grain cereal at breakfast. For lunch, a sandwich on whole-wheat bread. Dinner, a bowl of pasta topped with a tomato-based meat sauce.

How many servings of starches you need depends on your calorie needs. On the lighter end of the calorie scale, 6 servings of starches a day is recommended. On the heavier side of the calorie scale, 11 or more servings of starches a day is recommended. (See chart p. 294)

To some people that sounds like a lot. It's really not. For example, 8 servings of starches looks like this: 2 servings as 1 cup of cooked oatmeal at breakfast, 3 servings as a baked potato topped with bean chili for lunch, and 3 servings as 1 cup of pasta and a dinner roll at supper.

A serving of starch without added fat contains about 15 grams of carbohydrate, 3 grams of protein, and 80 calories. If you use the exchange system, that's the same as 1 starch exchange. In general, 1 serving is 1/2 cup grain, pasta, beans, or starchy vegetable; 1 ounce bread or dry cereal. For more specifics, see p. 83–86.

Grains

No major civilization has ever developed in the absence of a basic cereal grain. Ceres, the goddess of all vegetation and worshipped by the Romans, gives us our word "cereal."

Grains account for three-fourths of the world's food supply and are part of every culture. They are eaten whole (rice, oatmeal), as baked goods (bread, tortillas, crackers), and as pasta (spaghetti, couscous, spaetzle, udon noodles).

There are three parts to a grain. The germ is the center. It's rich in protein, poly-unsaturated fatty acids, vitamins, and minerals. The endosperm, the middle part, is mostly starch. The bran is the outer covering; it's rich in nutrients and fiber.

In their natural state, grains are chock full of B vitamins, iron, potassium, and fiber. However, grains are often refined. When refined, brown rice, for example, loses its bran to make white rice. Refined flours, such as white flour, are made from the endosperm only and have almost no fiber and decreased vitamins and minerals.

Wheat, White, Rye, or Pumpernickel?

When buying bread, you'll want ones made from whole grains, so you get the germ, the bran, and the endosperm. Look at the ingredient list. You want to see "whole-wheat flour" or a combination of whole-grain ingredients listed first.

"Whole-wheat" bread: This bread is made entirely from whole-grain wheat flour, which contains all the components of the wheat kernel: the germ, bran, and endosperm.

"Wheat" bread: This is not whole-wheat bread. Wheat bread usually contains a mixture of about 75 percent white flour and 25 percent whole-wheat flour.

It's sometimes hard to tell if the bread you're buying is made with whole-grain or whole-wheat flour. Don't be fooled! Not all brown bread is whole-wheat. The brown color may be from caramel coloring, which will be listed on the label. Its nutrient value is similar to white bread. Most store-purchased rye or pumpernickel bread is made mostly with white flour.

Likewise, choose crackers that are labeled "whole-wheat" or "whole-grain."

It's easier to pick out whole-grain pastas. Unlike some bread companies, manufacturers of white-flour pastas don't darken their pasta to make it look more "whole wheat." And just as with bread, whole-wheat pastas will be labeled as such.

You'll see "enriched" on many grain products. This means most of the nutrients that were lost during processing have been added back. When it comes to cereals and breads, often the B vitamins (thiamin, riboflavin, and niacin) and iron are added back. Other components of whole-grain products, such as antioxidants and fatty acids, are not added back.

You'll also see "fortified" on food labels. Fortified means vitamins or minerals that aren't found in the food naturally or found in only very small amounts are added to the food. More and more foods are fortified today. Folic acid is added to grain products, calcium is added to orange juice and cereals, milk is fortified with vitamin A and D, and in some areas, fat-free milk has extra calcium added.

THE WHOLE TRUTH ABOUT BAGELS

Years ago most people thought of bagels as a Jewish food, along with gefilte fish and chicken soup with matzo balls. Not so today! Bagels are everywhere from bagel shops to sandwich shops. Even the fast-food giants now offer bagels. Supermarkets carry them in the frozen section and the bakery aisle.

What's so great about bagels? They taste good, and most have no fat (before the cream cheese is added, that is).

But it's time for a reality check. Many people think of a bagel as no more calories and grams of carbohydrate than two slices of bread. Surprise! An average bagel, not even the largest New York bagel found on the streets of Manhattan, is equivalent to three to four slices of bread, or 45 to 60 grams of carbohydrate. No wonder people think bagels raise their blood glucose. If you think you're eating 30 grams of carbohydrate and you eat more in the range of 60 grams, your blood glucose will rise more than you expected.

Here are the nutrition facts from a few brands of bagels.

Bagel	Calories	Carbohydrate (g)	Exchanges/Servings
Bruegger's, Honey Grain	300	58	4 Starch
Dunkin Donuts, Pumpernickel	340	70	4 1/2 Starch
Lender's, Big and Crusty, Egg	230	47	3 Starch
Manhattan, Everything	290	54	3 1/2 Starch

Healthy Tips for Eating Bagels

- Check out the nutrition facts about the bagels you buy. If you buy supermarket bagels, the nutrition facts are on the label. If you buy bagels at a restaurant, ask for the nutrition facts there.
- Choose small bagels that have the lowest carbohydrate count unless you need a large amount of carbohydrate at one time.
- If you bring bagels home, cut them in half or thirds. Then eat either one-half or two-thirds at a time rather than the whole bagel.
- Use light cream cheese spreads and spread lightly. They still have a good bit of fat and calories.
- Consider opting for low-sugar jam or jelly rather than cream cheese, if fat and calories are a concern.

Whole Grains

When you eat whole grains, you get all the healthful parts of the grain—the fiber- and nutrient-rich bran, the endosperm, and the germ. You can get the goodness of whole grains starting first thing in the morning with a bowl of oatmeal. As for the rest of the day, take an idea from chefs in the finest of restaurants: Experiment with different grains. Most of the grains described below can be found in natural food stores and some major supermarkets. Buy in bulk to save money. Store in glass containers in the refrigerator or in a cool, dry place.

Amaranth: A staple of the Aztecs 8,000 years ago. It has very high-quality protein. Nutty flavor.

Barley: A staple in Tibet, China, and Japan. Used in the brewing industry. Barley is less nutritious when pearled, but pearled does take a shorter time to cook.

Buckwheat: It's really a fruit! Very good for people allergic to wheat. Roasted buckwheat is called kasha.

Corn: Also called maize. Popular in North and South America. Worshipped by many Indians. Ninety percent of the crop is fed to animals.

Millet: Used as an alternative to rice in many countries, especially China, India, and Africa. Very nutritious and the easiest grain to digest. Often used as a breakfast cereal.

Quinoa: Grown and revered by the Incas, quinoa (pronounced KEEN-wa) is being rediscovered! It has high-quality protein (all the essential amino acids) and is also high in calcium, iron, and fiber. Quinoa is higher in unsatu- rated fats and lower in carbohydrates than most other grains. Tiny and bead- shaped, it has a bit of a crunch to it with a light taste. Quinoa takes less time to cook than rice does.

Rice: A staple in China, Japan, and Africa. More rice is eaten than any other grain. It provides half the energy intake for 1.6 billion people. Brown rice still has its bran, so it's more nutri- tious than white rice.

Rye: Popular in Eastern Europe, Russia, and Scandinavia. It was con- sidered an unwanted seed for many centuries. It is the hardiest grain, often grown in cold climates and poor soils. It is similar to wheat nutritionally but has less gluten.

Wheat: A staple food for over half the world. Bulgur wheat and couscous are a form of cracked wheat.

Wild rice: Wild rice is actually a grass! Many people prefer wild rice over brown rice and fortunately wild rice is just as nutritious. It actually has more protein, riboflavin, and zinc than brown or white rice.

Grain Cookery

Boiling: Sprinkle one cup of the grain slowly into boiling water or fat-free, reduced-sodium chicken broth. Cover the pot with a tight-fitting lid so the grain gets the steam it needs to swell, lower the heat, and cook until the water is absorbed. Avoid the tendency to play chef here—don't stir while the grain cooks. If you do, the grain will come out a mushy mess! Set your kitchen timer for 10 minutes less than the usual cooking time. You can always cook it longer.

If you have trouble cooking grains, you may want to invest in a rice cooker. Who doesn't sometimes forget there is something on the stove until it is too late? A rice cooker shuts off when the rice or grain is cooked.

Sautéing: Add 1 Tbsp oil to a saucepan and sauté one cup grain for about 5 minutes to bring out the flavor. Then add the correct amount of water or broth, lower the heat, cover the pot with a tight-fitting lid, and cook until the water is absorbed.

Wheat Germ
toasted, unsweetened

How to Buy: Wheat germ is sold in both toasted and natural or raw forms. Many people prefer the toasted because it has a better flavor. Sold in bags, in bulk, and in jars. Found in most major supermarkets, usually in the cereal aisle.

How to Store: Store in the refrigerator or freezer. The unsaturated fats in wheat germ will go rancid if kept at room temperature. Will keep for about one year under refrigeration.

Uses: Sprinkle wheat germ on dry cereal, when making hot cereal, on salad, in casseroles. Bake into quick and yeast breads. Use like bread crumbs in meat loaf and patties.

> **EXCELLENT!**
>
> In the Nutrition Superstar descriptions, "excellent source of" means a serving of the food provides 20% or greater of the Daily Value (DV), or Recommended Dietary Allowance for that nutrient. "Good source of" means the food provides 10 to 19% of the DV for that nutrient.

Barley and Brown Rice in Many Ways

Serving Size: 1/2 cup, Total Servings: 6

Master Recipe

2 tsp olive oil

1 small onion, minced

1 stalk celery, minced

1 cup pearled barley or brown rice, rinsed

2 1/2 cups fat-free, reduced-sodium chicken broth

1 In a wide, heavy saucepan over medium-high heat, heat the oil. Add the onion and celery and sauté for 3 minutes. Add the barley or brown rice and sauté for 2 minutes.

2 Add the broth and bring to a boil. Lower the heat to simmer, cover, and cook for 40–45 minutes until barley or rice is tender.

Variations

Nutty

Add in 2 Tbsp toasted pine nuts, walnuts, or almonds after grain is cooked. Cook for 1 more minute.

Herb

Add in 1 Tbsp minced parsley, 2 tsp minced thyme, 1 tsp minced chives after grain is cooked.

Lemon Raisin

Add in 1 tsp grated lemon zest, 1 Tbsp fresh lemon juice, and 1/4 cup golden raisins after barley or rice is cooked. Cook 2 more minutes.

Tex Mex

Add in 1/2 cup diced tomatoes and 1/2 cup corn to barley or rice during the last 10 minutes of cooking. Finish cooking time.

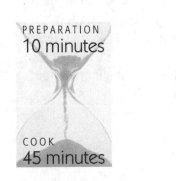

PREPARATION
10 minutes

COOK
45 minutes

Exchanges, Master Recipe
1 1/2 Starch

Calories 126
   Calories from Fat 18
Total Fat . . . . 2 g
   Saturated Fat . . . . 0 g
Cholesterol . . . . 0 mg
Sodium . . . . 208 mg
Carbohydrate . . . . 23 g
   Dietary Fiber . . . . 2 g
   Sugars . . . . 1 g
Protein . . . . 4 g

Nutty Blueberry Pancakes

Serving Size: 4 pancakes, Total Servings: 6

Splurge once in a while and skip the cereal. A pancake is a perfect canvas for adding so many nutritious foods. Here the wheat germ, sesame seeds, and blueberries all provide fiber, vitamins, and minerals. Make sure you buy toasted wheat germ and that the sesame seeds are also toasted to get a good nutty taste.

2 eggs	**1/4** cup toasted sesame seeds
1/4 cup canola oil	**3** Tbsp brown sugar
1 1/2 cups low-fat buttermilk	**1 1/2** tsp baking powder
1 cup all-purpose flour	**1/4** tsp salt
1/2 cup toasted wheat germ	**1** cup washed fresh blueberries

1 In a large bowl, beat together the eggs, oil, and buttermilk.

2 In a separate bowl, combine the flour, wheat germ, sesame seeds, brown sugar, baking powder, and salt.

3 Add the flour mixture to the egg mixture and mix until blended. Fold the blueberries into the batter.

4 Spray a nonstick griddle with nonstick spray. Heat the griddle for 1 minute over medium-high heat. Add the batter by tablespoons, 2 Tbsp per pancake. Cook on one side until edges are bubbly and look dry. Turn the pancakes over and cook for 2–3 minutes until pancake is golden brown. Repeat until batter is used up. Serve immediately.

PREPARATION
20 minutes

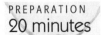

COOK
5-6 minutes

Exchanges
2 1/2 Starch
2 1/2 Fat

Calories 320
 Calories from Fat 143
Total Fat . . . . 16 g
 Saturated Fat . . . . 2 g
Cholesterol . . . . 73 mg
Sodium . . . . .278 mg
Carbohydrate . . . . .35 g
 Dietary Fiber . . . . .3 g
 Sugars . . . . 14 g
Protein . . . . 10 g

Couscous Many Ways

Serving Size: 1/2 cup, Total Servings: 6

Master Recipe

2 tsp olive oil

1 small onion, minced

1 cup dry couscous

1 1/2 cups fat-free, reduced-sodium chicken broth

Salt and pepper to taste

1 In a large, heavy skillet over medium-high heat, heat the oil. Add the onion and sauté for 5 minutes. Add the couscous and sauté for 1 minute.

2 Add the broth and bring to a boil. Cover and remove from the heat. Let stand for 5 minutes until couscous has absorbed the liquid. Season with salt and pepper.

Variations

Vegetable

Add 1 cup diced carrots and 1 cup sliced zucchini to the onions. Sauté for 10 minutes. Proceed with recipe.

Sweet

Pour 1 cup boiling water over 1/2 cup raisins to plump. Let stand for 10 minutes. Drain. Add to the cooked couscous.

Curry

Add 1 tsp curry powder, 1/4 tsp coriander, 1/4 tsp cumin, and 1/8 tsp crushed red pepper flakes to onion. Sauté for 5 minutes. Proceed with recipe.

Italian

Substitute 1 cup canned crushed tomatoes mixed with 1/2 cup water for the chicken broth. Add 1 Tbsp minced basil and 1/2 cup canned chickpeas to the cooked couscous. Cook 1 more minute.

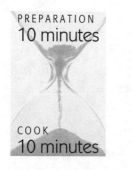

PREPARATION
10 minutes

COOK
10 minutes

Exchanges, Master Recipe

1 1/2 Starch

Calories 131
  Calories from Fat 14
Total Fat . . . . .2 g
  Saturated Fat . . . . .0 g
Cholesterol . . . . .0 mg
Sodium . . . . .123 mg
Carbohydrate . . . . .24 g
  Dietary Fiber . . . . .2 g
  Sugars . . . . .2 g
Protein . . . . .5 g

Basic Quinoa

Serving Size: 1/2 cup, Total Servings: 4

Quinoa is considered the supergrain of the future, but we think it is something you should try today! Quinoa is available in the grain section of most natural food and gourmet stores, but do check your local markets too.

1 cup quinoa

2 cups fat-free, reduced-sodium chicken broth

1/4 tsp ground black pepper

1 Using a fine sieve, rinse the quinoa several times with cool water. Rinsing the quinoa removes the bitter taste, called saponin, that quinoa holds in its outer ring. This is a very important step. Make sure you rinse the quinoa thoroughly.

2 In a saucepan over high heat, bring the broth to a boil. Slowly add the quinoa and bring to another boil. Lower the heat, cover, and simmer for 15 minutes until quinoa absorbs the broth.

3 Fluff with a fork and serve, or chill and use for cold salads.

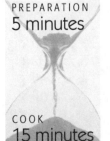

PREPARATION
5 minutes

COOK
15 minutes

Exchanges
2 Starch

Calories 150
 Calories from Fat 18
Total Fat . . . . .2 g
 Saturated Fat . . . . .0 g
Cholesterol . . . . .0 mg
Sodium . . . . .240 mg
Carbohydrate . . . . .25 g
 Dietary Fiber . . . . .4 g
 Sugars . . . . .0 g
Protein . . . . .7 g

Quinoa Stuffed Peppers

Serving Size: 1 pepper, Total Servings: 4

Quinoa is used here instead of ground beef as a stuffing for plump peppers. Try having the peppers cold the next day with a salad on the side. Try kidney, cannellini, or black beans in place of the chickpeas.

2 tsp olive oil	**1/2** cup cooked canned chickpeas, drained
1 small onion, minced	**2** Tbsp minced parsley
1 clove garlic, minced	**1** tsp dried thyme
1/2 cup diced celery	**1/2** tsp dried oregano
1/2 cup diced red pepper	Salt and pepper to taste
1/4 cup diced carrots	**4** large red or green peppers
1 cup quinoa, rinsed	
2 cups fat-free, reduced-sodium chicken broth	

1 In a skillet over medium-high heat, heat the oil. Add the onion and garlic and sauté for 2 minutes. Add the celery, peppers, and carrots and sauté for 5 minutes. Add the quinoa and sauté for 1 minute. Add the broth and bring to a boil. Lower the heat, cover, and simmer for 15 minutes until quinoa has absorbed the broth.

2 Add the chickpeas, parsley, thyme, oregano, salt, and pepper and mix well. Set aside. Preheat the oven to 350°F.

3 Slice the tops off the peppers and remove the seeds and as much of the white membrane as you can. Cut a small sliver off the bottom of each pepper so that it stands upright. Don't cut through or the quinoa filling will fall out.

4 Bring a stockpot of water filled 2/3 full to a boil. Add the peppers and boil for 4-5 minutes. Using tongs, remove the peppers and let cool for 10 minutes. Spoon some of the quinoa stuffing into each pepper. Place all the stuffed peppers standing upright in a casserole dish. Cover the peppers loosely with foil. Bake for 20-25 minutes until peppers are soft.

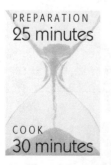

PREPARATION
25 minutes

COOK
30 minutes

Exchanges
2 Starch   1/2 Fat
3 Vegetable (or 1 Carbohydrate)

Calories 266	
Calories from Fat 45	
Total Fat . . . . 5 g	
Saturated Fat . . . . 1 g	
Cholesterol . . . . 0 mg	
Sodium . . . . 292 mg	
Carbohydrate . . . . 46 g	
Dietary Fiber . . . . 10 g	
Sugars . . . . 8 g	
Protein . . . . 10 g	

Quinoa Salad

Serving Size: about 1/2 cup, Total Servings: 4

Because of its mild flavor, quinoa makes a nice light salad. Stuff this salad into a hollowed out large tomato or long zucchini. If you want this hot, just sauté the vegetables in the olive oil, add to the cooked quinoa, add the vinegar, and serve.

1/2	cup raw quinoa, rinsed	**2**	Tbsp minced fresh parsley
1/4	cup finely chopped yellow pepper	**1 1/2**	Tbsp olive oil
1/4	cup finely chopped red pepper	**4**	Tbsp rice vinegar
1/4	cup finely chopped carrot	**2**	cloves garlic, minced
1/4	cup finely chopped celery	**2**	Tbsp minced green onions
			Fresh ground pepper and salt to taste

1 Prepare the quinoa. Rinse the quinoa in a fine sieve for 20 seconds. In a 1-quart saucepan bring 1 1/2 cups water to a boil. Add the quinoa and bring to a boil. Lower the heat to simmer, cover, and cook for 15 minutes.

2 Meanwhile prepare the vegetables. Combine the chopped yellow pepper, red pepper, carrot, celery, and parsley in a medium bowl.

3 In a blender, combine the oil, vinegar, garlic, green onions, salt, and pepper. Blend for 15 seconds.

4 Once the quinoa is cooked, add it to the vegetables. Pour the dressing over the quinoa and vegetables and toss well. Refrigerate for 1 hour. Serve over lettuce if desired.

PREPARATION
20 minutes

COOK
15 minutes

Exchanges
1 Starch
1 Fat

Calories 125
  Calories from Fat 51
Total Fat . . . . 6 g
  Saturated Fat . . . . 1 g
Cholesterol . . . . 0 mg
Sodium . . . . 12 mg
Carbohydrate . . . . 16 g
  Dietary Fiber . . . . 3 g
  Sugars . . . . 2 g
Protein . . . . 3 g

Basic Wild Rice
Serving Size: 1/2 cup, Total Servings: 6

1 cup wild rice

4 cups water

Salt and pepper to taste

1 Rinse the wild rice in several changes of water until the water runs clear. Wild rice is a grass, so there is often a small amount of debris in the rice.

2 Bring the water to a boil in a 3-quart saucepan. Slowly add the rice and bring to another boil. Lower the heat, cover, and simmer about 45 minutes to 1 hour until rice has absorbed the water.

PREPARATION
5 minutes

COOK
45 minutes to 1 hour

Exchanges
1 Starch

Calories 95
  Calories from Fat 3
Total Fat . . . . 0 g
  Saturated Fat . . . . 0 g
Cholesterol . . . . 0 mg
Sodium . . . . 2 mg
Carbohydrate . . . . 20 g
  Dietary Fiber . . . . 2 g
  Sugars . . . . 1 g
Protein . . . . 4 g

Wild Rice Salad

Serving Size: about 1 cup, Total Servings: 4

Wild rice tends to be a bit more expensive than other rices, but it's worth it. This salad is a nice change from hot cooked wild rice.

1 cup raw wild rice	**1** small shallot, minced
4 cups cold water	**1** tsp minced thyme
1 cup mandarin oranges, packed in their own juice. Drain, but reserve 2 Tbsp of the juice.	**2** Tbsp raspberry vinegar
	2 Tbsp olive oil
1/2 cup chopped celery	Fresh ground pepper and salt to taste
1/4 cup minced red pepper	

1 Prepare the rice: Rinse the raw rice in several changes of water until the water runs clear.

2 Put the raw rice and the 4 cups of water in a medium saucepan. Bring to a boil, lower the heat to low, cover, and simmer for 45 minutes to 1 hour, until the rice has absorbed the liquid. Set the rice aside to cool.

3 Meanwhile in a large bowl, combine the mandarin oranges, celery, red pepper, and shallot.

4 In a small bowl, combine the reserved mandarin orange juice, thyme, vinegar, and oil. Add the rice to the mandarin orange mixture.

5 Add the dressing and toss to coat. Refrigerate for 1 hour.

PREPARATION
25 minutes

COOK
50 minutes

Exchanges

2 Starch	1/2 Fruit
1 Fat	

Calories 231
   Calories from Fat 59
Total Fat . . . . 7 g
   Saturated Fat . . . . 1 g
Cholesterol . . . . 0 mg
Sodium . . . . 20 mg
Carbohydrate . . . . 39 g
   Dietary Fiber . . . . 4 g
   Sugars . . . . 7 g
Protein . . . . 7 g

Italian Wild Rice Pilaf

Serving Size: about 3/4 cup, Total Servings: 4

In parts of Italy, wild rice is as popular as the traditional arborio rice. This pilaf shines with little specks of sun-dried tomatoes, sweet dribbles of balsamic vinegar, all topped with the crunch of pine nuts. This is also good as a cold salad.

2 tsp olive oil	**1** recipe Basic Wild Rice
2 cloves garlic, minced	**2** Tbsp minced parsley
1 small onion, diced	**2** Tbsp balsamic vinegar
1/2 cup diced celery	**1** Tbsp toasted pine nuts
1 cup chopped rehydrated sun-dried tomatoes or 2 plum tomatoes, chopped	Salt and pepper to taste

1 In a skillet over medium-high heat, heat the oil. Add the garlic and onions and sauté for 5 minutes. Add the celery and sauté for 3 minutes. Add the sun-dried tomatoes or diced tomatoes and sauté for 3 minutes.

2 Add the cooked rice and cook 1 minute.

3 Add the vinegar, parsley, and pine nuts and cook for 1 minute more.

PREPARATION
15 minutes

COOK
15 minutes (plus 45 minutes to 1 hour to prepare rice)

Exchanges
2 Starch
1 Vegetable
1/2 Fat

Calories 198
   Calories from Fat 35
Total Fat . . . . 4 g
   Saturated Fat . . . . 1 g
Cholesterol . . . . 0 mg
Sodium . . . . 21 mg
Carbohydrate . . . . 36 g
   Dietary Fiber . . . . 4 g
   Sugars . . . . 5 g
Protein . . . . 7 g

Confetti Rice and Beans

Serving Size: about 3/4 cup, Total Servings: 6

This rice-and-bean dish is made even healthier with the addition of bell peppers, which are rich in vitamin C. The peppers add brilliant color. Substitute kidney beans for the black beans if you like.

2 tsp olive oil	1 cup canned black beans, drained
1 medium onion, diced	1/2 cup diced red pepper
2 cloves garlic, minced	1/2 cup diced yellow pepper
1 bay leaf	1/2 cup diced green pepper
1 cup long-grain white rice or basmati rice	1/2 tsp ground cumin
2 cups fat-free, reduced-sodium chicken broth	1/2 tsp ground coriander
	Salt and pepper to taste

1 In a saucepan over medium-high heat, heat the oil. Add the onion and garlic and sauté for 4 minutes. Add the bay leaf and rice and sauté for 2 minutes.

2 Add the broth and bring to a boil. Lower the heat, cover, and simmer for 15 minutes.

3 Add the beans and cook for 5 minutes. Add the peppers, cumin, and coriander and cook for 5 minutes. Add salt and pepper to taste.

PREPARATION
20 minutes

COOK
35 minutes

Exchanges
2 Starch
1 Vegetable

Calories 188
　Calories from Fat 16
Total Fat . . . . 2 g
　Saturated Fat . . . . 0 g
Cholesterol . . . . 0 mg
Sodium . . . . 200 mg
Carbohydrate . . . . 36 g
　Dietary Fiber . . . . 4 g
　Sugars . . . . 4 g
Protein . . . . 6 g

Basic Polenta

Serving Size: about 1/2 cup, Total Servings: 6

Master Recipe

1 cup whole-grain yellow cornmeal

2 cups water

2 cups 1% milk

Salt and pepper to taste

1 Mix the cornmeal with 1 cup of the water. Mix until smooth.

2 In a saucepan, bring the remaining 1 cup of water and the milk to a boil. Season with salt and pepper. Reduce the heat to medium and slowly add the cornmeal. Cook for 5 minutes over medium heat.

3 Lower the heat to very low and simmer the polenta while stirring frequently until the polenta pulls away from the sides of the pan, about 10–15 minutes.

4 Immediately serve as is or proceed to Grilled Polenta variation.

Flavor Variations

Herb

Add 2 Tbsp minced herb of choice.

Cheese

Add 2 Tbsp grated Parmesan cheese.

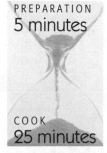

PREPARATION
5 minutes

COOK
25 minutes

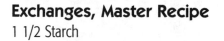

Exchanges, Master Recipe
1 1/2 Starch

Calories	126
Calories from Fat	18
Total Fat	2 g
Saturated Fat	0 g
Cholesterol	0 mg
Sodium	208 mg
Carbohydrate	23 g
Dietary Fiber	2 g
Sugars	1 g
Protein	4 g

Grilled Variation

1 After proceeding through step 3 of the master recipe, spread the polenta on a baking sheet that is 1/4-inch in depth. Put the pan in the refrigerator and chill at least 2 hours or overnight until the polenta is firm.

2 With a knife, cut the polenta into 6 wedges. Place the wedges on a broiler pan that has been sprayed with nonstick spray. Drizzle each polenta wedge with 1/2 tsp olive oil.

3 Broil the polenta squares 6 inches from the heat source for 1–2 minutes per side.

Toppings (for Master or Grilled Recipe)

1/4 cup low-fat, low-sodium marinara sauce (1/4 cup per serving)

  2 cups cooked sliced mushrooms (1/3 cup per serving)

  2 cups cooked diced zucchini (1/3 cup per serving)

Cranberry Rice
Serving Size: 1/2 cup, Total Servings: 4

Most people enjoy summer fruits more than winter ones. In some parts of the country in the winter, the choices for fruit are quite limited. Why not try a little dried fruit to boost your fruit consumption? Dried cranberries go well in grain dishes and add a beautiful jewel-like appearance. Try dried cherries or blueberries, too.

1 package wild and white rice   **1** tsp orange zest

1/4 cup toasted walnuts   **1** tsp olive oil

1/4 cup sliced green onions   Salt and pepper to taste

1/2 cup dried cranberries

1 Prepare the rice according to package directions (includes 1 Tbsp butter).

2 In a medium bowl, mix together the walnuts, green onions, cranberries, zest, olive oil, salt, and pepper. Add the rice and toss well.

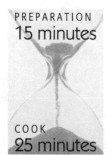

PREPARATION
15 minutes

COOK
25 minutes

Exchanges
2 Starch   1 Fruit
1 1/2 Fat

Calories 278
  Calories from Fat 83
Total Fat . . . . 9 g
  Saturated Fat . . . . 2 g
Cholesterol . . . . 7 mg
Sodium . . . . 502 mg
Carbohydrate . . . . 45 g
  Dietary Fiber . . . . 2 g
  Sugars . . . . 12 g
Protein . . . . 6 g

Pasta

When buying pastas, consider buying whole-wheat versions. Whole-wheat pasta has about 3 times the fiber, plus antioxidants and other nutrients not found in pasta made with white flour.

The colored pastas such as carrot, beet, or spinach are certainly pretty and add variety but they don't count as a vegetable serving (sorry!). Add real vegetables to your pasta dishes to get their nutrient content higher.

Keep your dry pastas in a cool, dry pantry. Use them within a year.

New Ways With Pasta

- Add peas, asparagus, chopped cauliflower, or sliced carrots during the last 3–4 minutes of the pasta cooking time. The pasta will absorb some of the vegetable flavor.

- Boil pasta in fat-free, reduced-sodium chicken broth, or broth plus a chopped onion or garlic clove.

- Top cooked pasta with

  - One of the new, reduced-fat cream soups for a tasty sauce.

  - Canned low-fat chili (2 Tbsp per serving) plus a sprinkle of low-fat cheese.

  - Heated salsa.

- Toss cooked pasta with a bit of olive oil and a can of water-packed tuna, drained. Top with a bit of Parmesan cheese.

- Thin bottled pesto sauce with fat-free, reduced-sodium chicken broth to lower the fat content. Toss in pasta and add chopped rehydrated sun-dried tomatoes.

- Add chopped ginger to pasta as it cooks; top pasta with lite soy sauce and a can of heated Asian vegetables.

- Add any kind of cooked dried or canned beans to the pasta to add non-animal protein to the dish.

Fusilli with Sage and Peppers

Serving Size: about 1 cup, Total Servings: 8

A dish made with peppers is not only healthy (more vitamin C than citrus!) but looks pretty too. Use the sauce over rice or a baked potato for a different topping.

1 1/2 Tbsp olive oil

1 medium onion, coarsely chopped

1/2 each of red, yellow, green, and orange peppers (try to find as many different peppers as you can, if you only have two or three, that is fine), cut into thin strips

3 cloves garlic, minced

1 Tbsp fresh sage, minced

1 1/2 cups canned tomato sauce

2 tsp tomato paste

2 Tbsp dry red wine

1/8 tsp red pepper flakes (Optional. Add if you want a little kick!)

Salt and pepper

1 pound fusilli, or other shaped pasta such as rigatoni or penne, cooked

1 In a large skillet over medium heat, heat the oil. Add the onion and sauté for 2 minutes. Add the garlic, peppers, and sage. Sauté for 3 more minutes.

2 Add the tomato sauce, tomato paste, and red wine. Bring to a boil, lower the heat, and let simmer for 10 minutes. Add the red pepper flakes, salt, and pepper. Pour the sauce on each portion of cooked fusilli.

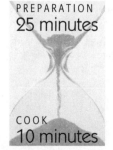

PREPARATION
25 minutes

COOK
10 minutes

Exchanges
3 Starch
1 Vegetable

Calories 262
  Calories from Fat 30
Total Fat . . . . 3 g
  Saturated Fat . . . . 1 g
Cholesterol . . . . 0 mg
Sodium . . . . 283 mg
Carbohydrate . . . . 50 g
  Dietary Fiber . . . . 4 g
  Sugars . . . . 6 g
Protein . . . . 8 g

Pasta Primavera

Serving Size: 1 cup pasta with sauce, Total Servings: 6

A cornucopia of vegetables in a creamy pasta dish. You can add broccoli, cauliflower, snow peas, spinach, or tomatoes. You are limited only by your imagination. The cream sauce can be used to top cooked poultry or pour over rice.

1 Tbsp plus 1 tsp olive oil	1 cup sliced red pepper
4 tsp flour	1/2 cup asparagus tips
1 1/2 cups 1% milk	2 Tbsp Parmesan cheese
1 cup low-fat ricotta cheese	6 cups cooked fettucine
1/2 cup chopped onion	2 Tbsp minced parsley
1 cup sliced carrots	

1 In a skillet over medium-high heat, heat 1 Tbsp of the oil. Add the flour and cook, stirring for 1 minute until flour is absorbed into the oil.

2 Remove the pan from the heat. Add in the milk slowly, whisking so that no lumps form. Return the pan to the heat and continue to cook until thickened. Add the ricotta cheese a little at a time, stirring after each addition, and remove from the heat.

3 In another skillet, heat remaining 1 tsp of oil. Add the carrots and sauté for 2–3 minutes. Add the red pepper and sauté for 2 minutes. Add the asparagus and cover and cook for 2 minutes.

4 Add the vegetables to the sauce and return to the heat. Add the Parmesan cheese and cook over low heat for 1 minute. Toss the cooked fettucine and sauce together. Sprinkle with parsley and serve.

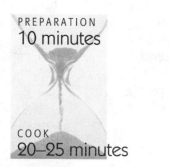

PREPARATION
10 minutes

COOK
20–25 minutes

Exchanges

2 1/2 Starch	1 Lean Meat
1 Vegetable	1/2 Fat

Calories 294	
Calories from Fat 67	
Total Fat . . . . 7 g	
Saturated Fat . . . . 3 g	
Cholesterol . . . . 62 mg	
Sodium . . . . 160 mg	
Carbohydrate . . . . 43 g	
Dietary Fiber . . . . 3 g	
Sugars . . . . 8 g	
Protein . . . . 16 g	

Penne Pasta with Basil Vinaigrette

Serving Size: 1 cup pasta, Total Servings: 4

The nutritional highlight of this salad is the plum tomatoes. Rich in vitamin C, tomatoes also boast a substantial amount of lycopene, another cancer-fighting agent. If you prefer to cook the tomatoes, we've given you the directions below.

2 lbs fresh plum tomatoes, seeded and cut into 1/2 inch cubes

1/4 cup olive oil

1/4 cup fresh chopped basil leaves

2 Tbsp balsamic vinegar

1/2 lb penne noodles

1/2 cup chopped red onion

1/2 cup chopped jarred roasted red peppers

Salt and pepper to taste

1 Combine the tomatoes, olive oil, basil, vinegar, pepper, and salt in a large serving bowl.

2 Meanwhile, cook the pasta in a large pot of boiling water until firm, about 8–9 minutes. Drain.

3 Combine the cooked pasta with the tomato mixture. Add the red onion and roasted red peppers. Serve at room temperature.

To have the tomatoes cooked: Combine the tomatoes, olive oil, basil, vinegar, salt, and pepper in a large skillet. Cook over medium heat until mixture boils. Lower the heat and simmer for 10 minutes. Add the cooked penne noodles, onions, and roasted peppers. Serve at once.

PREPARATION
20 minutes

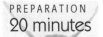

COOK
15 minutes for cooked version

Exchanges
3 Starch
2 Vegetable
2 Fat

Calories 369
   Calories from Fat 122
Total Fat . . . . 14 g
   Saturated Fat . . . . 3 g
Cholesterol . . . . 0 mg
Sodium . . . . 83 mg
Carbohydrate . . . . 54 g
   Dietary Fiber . . . . 4 g
   Sugars . . . . 10 g
Protein . . . . 9 g

Asian Noodle Salad

Serving Size: about 1 cup, Total Servings: 4

Instead of take-out sesame noodles, make your own. The peanut sauce is an all-around sauce that can be used on cooked chicken, beef, pork, or seafood. Or use the peanut sauce to top cooked vegetables such as carrots, asparagus, broccoli, or peppers.

4 cups thin spaghetti or udon noodles

1 cup slivered carrots

1/2 cup slivered celery

1/4 cup minced shallot

Dressing

1/3 cup reduced-fat peanut butter

3/4 cup fat-free, reduced-sodium chicken broth

2 Tbsp tamari soy sauce

1 tsp minced ginger

2 cloves garlic, minced

2 tsp arrowroot

1 Tbsp water

Crushed red pepper flakes

1 Tbsp minced cilantro

1 1/3 Tbsp black sesame seeds (found in the Asian sections of grocery stores)

4 cups salad greens of choice

1 In a salad bowl, combine the cooked noodles with the carrots, celery, and shallot.

2 In a small saucepan over medium-high heat, melt the peanut butter with the broth, soy sauce, ginger, and garlic. When mixture is boiling, combine the arrowroot and water. Add to the sauce. Cook until thickened.

3 Add the red pepper flakes and cilantro. Pour over the noodles and sprinkle with black sesame seeds. Chill for 1 hour. Serve over any greens of choice.

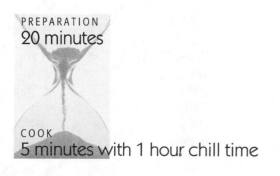

PREPARATION
20 minutes

COOK
5 minutes with 1 hour chill time

Exchanges

4 Starch	1 Vegetable
1 Fat	

Calories 382
   Calories from Fat 91
Total Fat . . . . .10 g
   Saturated Fat . . . . 2 g
Cholesterol . . . . 0 mg
Sodium . . . . 755 mg
Carbohydrate . . . . 64 g
   Dietary Fiber . . . . 7 g
   Sugars . . . . 10 g
Protein . . . . 15 g

Oven-dried Tomatoes, Garlic, and Pasta

Serving Size: 1 cup pasta, 2 tomatoes, Total Servings: 4

When Robyn was in France for a vacation several years ago, these oven-dried tomatoes were served in some of the finer restaurants. So intrigued by their deep rich flavor, she got the recipe. Even though the drying process takes 4 hours, you can be busy doing other things.

8 plum tomatoes	**2** Tbsp dry white wine
1 Tbsp plus 1 tsp olive oil	**4** cups cooked linguine
1/4 tsp kosher salt	**1/2** cup minced parsley
4 sprigs fresh thyme	Salt and pepper to taste
3 cloves garlic, minced	

1 Preheat the oven to 250°F. Cut a small X in the bottom of each plum tomato. Bring a large pot of water to a boil. Drop the tomatoes in the water and leave them in for 30 seconds. Drain and splash with cold water. Peel the tomatoes.

2 Cut each tomato in half and scoop out the seeds. Discard the seeds. Place the tomato halves on a baking sheet. Drizzle with olive oil and salt. Place the thyme sprigs on top. Bake the tomatoes for 4 hours until the tomatoes are semi-dry.

3 Remove the tomatoes from the oven and slice into strips and place in a large bowl.

4 In a small skillet over medium heat, heat remaining 1 tsp oil. Add the garlic and sauté for 30 seconds. Add the wine and cook 30 seconds more.

5 Add the garlic to the tomatoes. Toss in the cooked linguine. Top with parsley and season with salt and pepper.

PREPARATION
15 minutes

COOK
4 hours

Exchanges
2 1/2 Starch   1 Vegetable
1 Fat

Calories 263
   Calories from Fat 48
Total Fat . . . . 5 g
   Saturated Fat . . . . 1 g
Cholesterol . . . . 0 mg
Sodium . . . . 160 mg
Carbohydrate . . . . 45 g
   Dietary Fiber . . . . 3 g
   Sugars . . . . 5 g
Protein . . . . 8 g

Asian Scallop Fettucine

Serving Size: 3 ounces scallops, 1 cup pasta, Total Servings: 4

Fresh scallops are a real treat. Scallops should have an ocean-fresh smell and look plump and juicy. Cook them only to obtain a nice crust on the outside, but don't overcook them, or they will remind you of a little rubber ball!

1 Tbsp flour	1 Tbsp minced green onions
1/8 tsp salt	2 tsp lemon juice
Pepper to taste	1 tsp cornstarch or arrowroot
1 pound sea scallops	2 Tbsp dry white wine
1 Tbsp olive oil	1/4 cup fat-free, reduced-sodium chicken broth
2 cloves garlic, minced	
1 tsp minced ginger	4 cups cooked fettucine

1 In a zippered plastic bag, combine the flour, salt, and pepper. Lightly coat each scallop with the flour mixture and put on a plate.

2 In a skillet over medium-high heat, heat the oil. Add the garlic, ginger, and green onions and sauté for 2 minutes. Raise the heat to high and sauté the scallops for 2–3 minutes until scallops are browned but tender.

3 Combine the lemon juice, cornstarch, white wine, and broth. Add to the pan and cook for 1 minute.

4 Toss the scallops with the cooked fettucine.

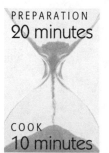

PREPARATION
20 minutes

COOK
10 minutes

Exchanges
2 Starch
2 Lean Meat

Calories 274
   Calories from Fat 51
Total Fat . . . . 6 g
   Saturated Fat . . . . 1 g
Cholesterol . . . . 70 mg
Sodium . . . . 269 mg
Carbohydrate . . . . 34 g
   Dietary Fiber . . . . 2 g
   Sugars . . . . 2 g
Protein . . . . 20 g

Angel Hair with Feta and Capers

Serving Size: 1 cup pasta, Total Servings: 4

One of our simplest pasta preparations with a big, bold taste. If you can, buy feta cheese from a specialty cheese shop rather than your supermarket. Not only will you have many more varieties to choose from, but the feta will be less salty. Good feta has a mild salty flavor that does not overpower.

2 tsp olive oil	**1/2** cup crumbled feta cheese
1 clove garlic, minced	**2** tsp capers
1 small tomato, seeded and diced	**1/2** tsp lemon zest
1 tsp minced fresh oregano	**4** cups cooked angel-hair pasta

1 In a skillet over medium heat, heat the oil. Add the garlic and tomato and sauté for 2 minutes. Add the oregano and sauté for 1 minute. Add the feta, capers, and lemon zest. Remove from heat.

2 Toss feta mixture with the angel hair and serve.

PREPARATION
10 minutes

COOK
10 minutes

Exchanges
3 Starch
1 Fat

Calories 272
   Calories from Fat 63
Total Fat . . . . 7 g
   Saturated Fat . . . . 3 g
Cholesterol . . . . 17 mg
Sodium . . . . 256 mg
Carbohydrate . . . . 42 g
   Dietary Fiber . . . . 2 g
   Sugars . . . . 4 g
Protein . . . . 11 g

Chicken, Spinach, and Shell Soup

Serving Size: about 1 1/4 cups, Total Servings: 4

Feeling a little under the weather? You are sure of a quick recovery with this soup. Not sick? You'll have a tasty soup to add to your winter meal repertoire.

2 tsp olive oil

1 small onion, chopped

2 cloves garlic, minced

1/2 lb fresh spinach, washed and chopped

3 cups fat-free, reduced-sodium chicken broth

1 cup whole tomatoes, drained and chopped

1/2 lb boneless, skinless chicken breasts, cut into 1/2-inch pieces

1 cup cooked small shell macaroni

Salt and pepper to taste

4 Tbsp grated Parmesan cheese

1 In a large pot over medium-high heat, heat the oil. Add the onion and garlic and sauté for 4 minutes. Add the spinach and cook for 2 minutes until spinach is wilted. Add the broth and tomatoes and bring to a boil. Lower the heat and simmer 15 minutes.

2 Add the chicken and simmer for 5 minutes more until chicken is cooked through.

3 Add the cooked shells and season with salt and pepper. Top each soup bowl with Parmesan cheese.

PREPARATION
20 minutes

COOK
20 minutes

Exchanges
1 Starch
2 Lean Meat
1 Vegetable

Calories 214
    Calories from Fat 56
Total Fat . . . . 6 g
    Saturated Fat . . . . 2 g
Cholesterol . . . . 42 mg
Sodium . . . . 641 mg
Carbohydrate . . . . 18 g
    Dietary Fiber . . . . 2 g
    Sugars . . . . 5 g
Protein . . . . 22 g

TWO ALL-TIME FAVORITE SAUCES FOR PASTA

Both of these sauces can be used time after time to create a quick, delicious dinner. Add vegetables, any kind of protein, or herbs and spices to create many variations. Both sauces can be frozen.

Marinara Sauce

Serving Size: 1/2 cup,
Total Servings: 6

- **2** tsp olive oil
- **2** cloves garlic, minced
- **1** small onion, diced
- **1** (16-oz) can tomatoes, with their liquid
- **1** (6-oz) can tomato paste
- **2** tsp sugar
- **2** Tbsp minced fresh basil
  Salt and pepper to taste

1 In a medium saucepan over medium heat, heat the oil. Add the garlic and onion and sauté for 3 minutes.

2 Add the remaining ingredients and bring to a boil. Lower the heat and simmer, uncovered, for 20 minutes until thick.

Exchanges
1 Carbohydrate

Calories 62	
Calories from Fat 16	
Total Fat . . . . .2 g	
Saturated Fat . . . . .0 g	
Cholesterol . . . . .0 mg	
Sodium . . . . .133 mg	
Carbohydrate . . . . .12 g	
Dietary Fiber . . . . .2 g	
Sugars . . . . .5 g	
Protein . . . . .2 g	

Pesto Sauce

Serving Size: 2 Tbsp,
Total Servings: 4

- **2** Tbsp olive oil
- **1/4** cup Parmesan cheese
- **1** cup fresh, chopped basil
- **1/4** cup fat-free, reduced-sodium chicken broth
- **3** cloves garlic, minced
- **1** Tbsp toasted pine nuts

1 Blend all ingredients in a blender at medium speed until well blended.

Exchanges
2 Fat

Calories 105	
Calories from Fat 86	
Total Fat . . . . .10 g	
Saturated Fat . . . . .3 g	
Cholesterol . . . . .8 mg	
Sodium . . . . .158 mg	
Carbohydrate . . . . .2 g	
Dietary Fiber . . . . .1 g	
Sugars . . . . .1 g	
Protein . . . . .4 g	

Beans, Peas, and Lentils

A Bonanza of Benefits

Legumes are also in the starch group. Legumes include beans, peas, and lentils. (We mean beans such as kidney, garbanzo, and white beans, not green or wax beans.)

They are all Nutrition Superstars.

- They are a good source of carbohydrate, and they raise blood glucose more slowly than some other carbohydrates.

- Legumes are a good source of protein without the fat and cholesterol of animal sources of protein.

- They are all excellent sources of fiber.

- They provide loads of vitamins (folate, thiamin, riboflavin, and niacin) and minerals (iron, zinc, phosphorus, and magnesium). Kidney beans, for example, are an excellent source of folate and a good source of magnesium, phosphorus, and copper. Lentils are also an excellent source of folate and a good source of iron, phosphorus, and copper.

- Dry legumes are very low in sodium. (Canned beans can contain a good bit of sodium. Rinse them to reduce the sodium.)

- Canned beans can be at-the-ready on your pantry shelf. Heat and eat them; toss them into soups, stews, sauces, casseroles, or salads; or blend them for dips or spreads.

- Legumes are a bargain. You won't find a less expensive source of great nutrition.

A half-cup of cooked beans, dried peas, or lentils has about 15 to 20 grams of carbohydrate and 5 to 10 grams of protein. Thus 1/2 cup counts as 1 starch exchange and 1 very lean meat exchange.

How to Buy: Beans, peas, and lentils come in dried form in either bags or boxes. Beans also come already cooked and ready to use in cans. Select cans that are neither rusted nor bulging.

PEAS: THE LITTLE LUXURY

Reportedly, Thomas Jefferson's contemporaries considered young fresh garden peas an exotic luxury, something like truffles today. Consider the pea more than a luxury but a sure-fire, nutrient-rich vegetable to include on the summer dining table.

The peak season for peas is May through August. Look for bright-green, crisp, well-filled pods. Refrigerate the peas in their pods and use as soon as possible. Shell the peas and cook in a small amount of water for 10 minutes until tender.

- Cook peas with finely chopped ginger. Add a dash of soy sauce when serving.
- Snip fresh mint or tarragon into the cooked peas, add just a drizzle of olive oil, and serve.
- Mix peas with cooked rice and add some fresh snipped chives and thyme.
- Mix cooked, cold corn and peas together, add shredded carrots and finely chopped shallot. Drizzle with red wine vinegar and olive oil for a delightful summer salad.

How to Store: Store dried beans in an airtight container in a cool, dry place for up to one year. Store canned beans in the pantry for up to one year.

Uses: Add to salads, soups, stews, and spreads.

If you have excess gas after you eat beans, here are two tricks to use. There is a digestive aid on the market called Beano. You put a drop or two into your bean dish. It really works! You can also drop a piece of seaweed such as kombu (available at health food stores or Oriental markets) into the cooking liquid.

How to Cook: You can use cooked, canned beans. Rinse them to reduce the sodium. Or you can cook dried beans yourself. You aren't personally involved in the process, so although they take time to soak and cook, you can be doing other things!

There are two ways to soak beans, a long way and a short way. Use the regular soaking method when you have time on your hands to soak beans. Use the quick soak method when you want beans in a hurry. (Split peas and lentils don't need soaking.)

Regular soak: Rinse beans with cool water and drain. Place beans in a large pot (any kind except unlined aluminum) with two to three times their volume of water and let stand for about 8 hours. If soaking time will be more than 12 hours, refrigerate beans during soaking to prevent fermentation.

Quick soak: Place the rinsed, drained beans in a pot with two to three times their volume of water. Bring to a boil, simmer for two minutes, cover, remove from heat, and let stand for one to two hours. Be sure to allow room in the pot for expansion, since dried beans will triple in volume during cooking.

Cooking: Cooking is the same after either method: Drain water. Add fresh water to beans and bring to a boil, keeping heat low, until tender. Use the timetable below for cooking times. For split peas, lentils, and other beans that don't require soaking, just add two to three times their volume of water and cook as for soaked beans.

	COOK TIME
Black beans	1 1/2–2 hours
Black-eyed peas	1 1/2–2 hours
Chickpeas	1 1/2–2 hours
Fava beans	2–3 hours
Kidney beans	1 1/2–2 hours
Lentils	45 minutes
Lima beans	45 minutes
Navy and pea beans	1 1/2–2 hours
Pinto beans	1 1/2–2 hours
Small pink beans	1 1/2–2 hours
Soybeans	3–3 1/2 hours
Split peas	45 minutes
White beans	1 1/2–2 hours

Almond-Pesto White Beans with Vegetables

Serving Size: about 3/4 cup, Total Servings: 4

We usually think of pesto as a topping for pasta, but over beans it works very well. Our pesto has a bit of a difference: We use almonds instead of the traditional pine nuts. Almonds have more calcium and overall are a good choice for nuts. The pesto can be made and frozen in zippered plastic bags. Just remove and defrost before using. You can use the pesto over rice, too.

Pesto

2 cloves garlic, minced

1 cup packed chopped basil

1/4 cup toasted slivered almonds

2 Tbsp Parmesan cheese

3 Tbsp olive oil

1 Tbsp fat-free, reduced-sodium chicken broth

1 tsp lemon juice

Salt and pepper to taste

1 tsp olive oil

White Beans and Vegetables

1/2 cup diced red onion

1 clove garlic, minced

1/2 cup diced carrot

1/2 cup diced zucchini, unpeeled

1 cup halved cherry tomatoes

2 cups canned white navy beans, drained

1 To make the pesto: Put the garlic, basil, almonds, and cheese in a food processor or blender and blend for a few seconds on high speed. Slowly add the oil, broth, and lemon juice, scraping down the sides of the food processor bowl or blender. Add salt and pepper to taste and set aside.

2 To prepare the white beans and vegetables: In a skillet over medium-high heat, heat the oil. Add the onion and garlic and sauté for 1 minute. Add the carrot and sauté for 3 minutes. Add the zucchini and cherry tomatoes and sauté for 3 minutes.

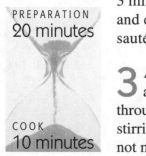

PREPARATION
20 minutes

COOK
10 minutes

3 Add in the white beans and pesto and heat through, about 1–2 minutes, stirring carefully so as to not mash the beans.

Exchanges

2 Starch   1 Very Lean Meat
1 Vegetable   2 Fat

Calories 307	
Calories from Fat 141	
Total Fat . . . . .16 g	
Saturated Fat . . . . 3 g	
Cholesterol . . . . 4 mg	
Sodium . . . . 279 mg	
Carbohydrate . . . . 32 g	
Dietary Fiber . . . . 9 g	
Sugars . . . . 7 g	
Protein . . . . .12 g	

Bow Tie Pasta with Sun-dried Tomato Pesto and White Beans

Serving Size: 1 1/2 cups, Total Servings: 8

This dish not only makes one of the most filling meals but it packs an extra boost of fiber from the addition of beans. If you can't find bow ties, substitute any shaped pasta you like.

2 cups boiling water

1 cup sun-dried tomatoes, rehydrated (Don't buy the sun-dried tomatoes in oil.)

1 lb bow tie noodles

1/4 cup fat-free ricotta cheese

1 Tbsp pine nuts, toasted (To toast: Put nuts in a dry skillet, and over medium heat shake the pan until the nuts are lightly toasted. Watch care fully so the nuts don't burn.)

1 Tbsp olive oil

1/4 cup chopped fresh basil

2 Tbsp chopped Italian parsley

1 Tbsp freshly grated Parmesan cheese

Salt and pepper to taste

2 cups cooked white beans (cannelini or navy beans)

Italian parsley for garnish

1 In a medium bowl, pour boiling water over the sun-dried tomatoes. Let stand for 15 minutes. Meanwhile, cook the bow tie noodles according to package directions (no added salt).

2 Drain the tomatoes. Chop the tomatoes into small pieces.

3 In a blender or food processor combine the tomatoes, ricotta cheese, olive oil, nuts, basil, parsley, Parmesan cheese, salt, and pepper until well blended.

4 In a saucepan combine the cooked white beans and pesto and heat until warmed throughout. To serve: On each plate, place the cooked bow ties first, top with beans mixed with pesto. Garnish with parsley.

PREPARATION
25 minutes

COOK (PASTA)
10 minutes

Exchanges

3 Starch   1 Vegetable

Calories 265
   Calories from Fat 31
Total Fat . . . . 3 g
   Saturated Fat . . . . 1 g
Cholesterol . . . . 3 mg
Sodium . . . . 20 mg
Carbohydrate . . . . 47 g
   Dietary Fiber . . . . 5 g
   Sugars . . . . 6 g
Protein . . . . 12 g

Colorful Lentil Salad

Serving Size: about 3/4 cup, Total Servings: 4

Lentils get dressed up in this bright salad. Perfect for barbecues and picnics as a replacement for the high-fat, low-fiber potato and macaroni salads.

2 cups cooked lentils

1/2 cup diced red pepper

1/2 cup diced green pepper

1/2 cup diced, seeded, peeled cucumber

2 celery stalks, washed and diced

1 small red onion, diced

2 cloves garlic, minced

2 Tbsp olive oil

2 tsp ground cumin

1/2 tsp dried oregano

3 Tbsp fresh lemon juice

Salt and pepper to taste

1 In a large salad bowl, combine the cooked lentils, red pepper, green pepper, cucumber, celery, and red onion.

2 In a blender or by hand in a bowl using a wire whisk combine the garlic, olive oil, ground cumin, oregano, lemon juice, salt, and pepper. Blend or whisk for 15 seconds. Pour the dressing over the salad. Refrigerate the salad for 1 hour.

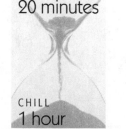

PREPARATION
20 minutes

CHILL
1 hour

Exchanges
1 1/2 Starch
1 Vegetable
1 Fat

Calories 198
　Calories from Fat 60
Total Fat . . . . 7 g
　Saturated Fat . . . . 1 g
Cholesterol . . . . 0 mg
Sodium . . . . 33 mg
Carbohydrate . . . . 27 g
　Dietary Fiber . . . . 10 g
　Sugars . . . . 5 g
Protein . . . . 10 g

Pasta Fagioli

Serving Size: 1 cup, Total Servings: 8

Fagioli means beans in Italian. No wonder the people of the Mediterranean are so healthy. Beans, vegetables, pasta, and olive oil all meld together in a mélange of flavors and nutrients. Pasta fagioli is similar to minestrone but thicker. This freezes beautifully. Just put the contents into a heavy freezer zippered plastic bag and freeze for up to 4 months.

1 Tbsp olive oil	4 cups fat-free, reduced-sodium chicken broth
3 cups chopped onions	2 cans (16-oz each) white cannellini or navy beans, rinsed and drained
4 cloves garlic, minced	
2 medium carrots, diced	2/3 cup minced rehydrated sun-dried tomatoes
2 medium zucchini, sliced	1/2 cup minced parsley
2 bay leaves	1/2 lb rigatoni or medium shells (any variety), cooked
1 Tbsp fresh basil	
1 Tbsp fresh oregano	Salt and pepper to taste
1 can (32-oz) crushed tomatoes	Crushed red pepper to taste

1 In a large skillet over medium heat, heat the oil. Add the onions and garlic and sauté for 5 minutes. Add the carrots and zucchini and sauté for 5 minutes.

2 Add the bay leaf, basil, oregano, broth, tomatoes, and beans. Cook until the vegetables are tender, about 10–15 minutes.

3 Add the sun-dried tomatoes, parsley, and pasta and cook for 5–10 minutes more. Season with salt, pepper, and crushed red pepper.

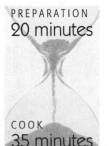

PREPARATION
20 minutes

COOK
35 minutes

Exchanges

3 Starch
4 Vegetable
(Or 4 Starch + 1 Vegetable)

Calories 336
　Calories from Fat 27
Total Fat . . . . 3 g
　Saturated Fat . . . . 0 g
Cholesterol . . . . 0 mg
Sodium . . . . 734 mg
Carbohydrate . . . . 63 g
　Dietary Fiber . . . . 11 g
　Sugars . . . . 16 g
Protein . . . . 16 g

Bean Salad in Many Ways

Serving Size: about 3/4 cup, Total Servings: 4

Beans are like a blank canvas. They take on the flavor of whatever you add to them, so you can increase your taste options. Here we've given you a basic format to follow to prepare bean salad. Then with a twist here and a tweak there, you can use this bean salad often without ever tiring of it.

Master Recipe

2 cups canned beans of choice, rinsed and drained

1/3 cup minced onion

1 clove garlic, minced

1/2 cup chopped celery

1/2 cup chopped carrot

1/2 cup seeded, diced tomato

2 Tbsp white wine vinegar

3 Tbsp olive oil

1 tsp lemon juice

Salt and pepper to taste

1 In a medium salad bowl, combine all ingredients. Cover and chill for 1/2 hour before serving.

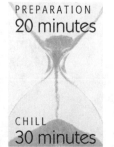

PREPARATION
20 minutes

CHILL
30 minutes

Exchanges, Master Recipe
1 1/2 Starch
1 Vegetable
2 Fat

Calories	226
Calories from Fat	95
Total Fat	11 g
Saturated Fat	2 g
Cholesterol	0 mg
Sodium	137 mg
Carbohydrate	26 g
Dietary Fiber	8 g
Sugars	6 g
Protein	8 g

Variations

Mexican

Use red kidney, black, or pinto beans. Add 1 Tbsp minced cilantro. Substitute red wine vinegar and lime juice for the white wine vinegar and lemon juice. Add 1/4 tsp chili powder.

Italian

Use chickpeas or cannellini beans. Add 1 Tbsp each minced Italian parsley and basil. Substitute balsamic vinegar for the white wine vinegar.

Asian

Use adzuki beans. Add 1 Tbsp minced cilantro. Substitute 2 Tbsp minced shallots for the onion. Substitute rice vinegar and sesame oil for the white wine vinegar and olive oil. Add 2 tsp toasted sesame seeds. Substitute 1/2 cup seeded, peeled, diced cucumber for the tomato.

French

Use Great Northern beans. Add 1 tsp Dijon mustard. Substitute champagne vinegar for the white wine vinegar. Add 1 tsp minced thyme. Substitute 1/4 cup minced green onions for the onion.

Indian

Use chickpeas. Add 1/2 tsp curry powder, 1/4 tsp cumin, and a dash of chili powder. Omit vinegar and increase lemon juice to 2 Tbsp. Use canola oil instead of olive oil.

Black Bean Jicama Salad

Serving Size: about 1 cup, Total Servings: 8

Jicama, the Mexican potato, is one of my favorite vegetables. It is a brown-skinned vegetable the size of an orange to the size of a football. To use, you just peel the skin off and cut slices. It has a texture like a water chestnut, is slightly sweet, and is low in calories. It is my personal promise that this salad will disappear from everyone's plate fast, so make a lot!

3 cups cooked black beans (from scratch; or canned, rinsed, and drained)

2 tomatoes, chopped

1 cup diced jicama

2 red peppers, finely chopped

1 cup yellow corn (off the cob or frozen)

3 jalapeño peppers, chopped (for a slightly less hot taste, remove the seeds)

3 cloves garlic, minced

2 Tbsp fresh chopped cilantro

1 Tbsp cumin

1 Tbsp olive oil

3 Tbsp lime juice

1 Tbsp red wine vinegar

Salt and pepper to taste

1 In a large salad bowl, combine all ingredients. Cover and refrigerate for at least 2 hours.

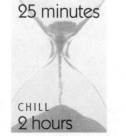

PREPARATION
25 minutes

CHILL
2 hours

Exchanges

1 1/2 Starch
1 Vegetable

Calories 146
   Calories from Fat 20
Total Fat . . . . .2 g
   Saturated Fat . . . . .0 g
Cholesterol . . . . .0 mg
Sodium . . . . 90 mg
Carbohydrate . . . . .27 g
   Dietary Fiber . . . . .8 g
   Sugars . . . . .5 g
Protein . . . . .7 g

Spanish Black Bean Soup
Serving Size: 1 cup, Total Servings: 6

2 tsp chicken broth

1 tsp olive oil

3 cloves garlic, minced

1 medium yellow onion, minced

1 tsp fresh minced oregano

1 tsp cumin

1 tsp chili powder or 1/2 tsp cayenne pepper

1 medium red pepper, chopped

1 medium carrot, coarsely chopped

3 cups cooked black beans (from scratch; or canned, rinsed, and drained)

1 1/2 cups fat-free, reduced-sodium chicken broth

1/2 cup dry red wine

Salt and pepper to taste

1 In a large stockpot, over medium-high heat, heat the 2 tsp chicken broth and 1 tsp oil. Add the garlic and onions and sauté for 3 minutes. Add the oregano, cumin, and chili powder and stir for another minute. Add the red pepper and carrot and sauté for 2 minutes.

2 Puree 1 1/2 cups of the black beans in a blender or food processor. Add the pureed beans to the pot. Add the remaining 1 1/2 cups of the whole beans, chicken broth, and red wine. Simmer and let cook for 1 hour. Season with salt and pepper.

PREPARATION
20 minutes

COOK
1 hour

Exchanges
1 1/2 Starch
1 Very Lean Meat

Calories 149
    Calories from Fat 12
Total Fat . . . . .1 g
    Saturated Fat . . . . .0 g
Cholesterol . . . . .0 mg
Sodium . . . . .134 mg
Carbohydrate . . . . .26 g
    Dietary Fiber . . . . .9 g
    Sugars . . . . .5 g
Protein . . . . .9 g

White Bean Chili

Serving Size: 1 cup, Total Servings: 6

We usually think of chili as red in color. White beans such as navy or cannellini beans give an interesting twist to traditional chili.

1 Tbsp olive oil	2 1/2 cups fat-free, reduced-sodium chicken broth
1 medium onion, chopped	
3 cloves garlic, minced	3 cups cooked white navy beans or cannelini beans
3 Tbsp minced green pepper	1 cup white corn (frozen or fresh)
2 Tbsp unbleached white flour	Salt and pepper to taste
1 Tbsp ground cumin	Garnish: 1/4 cup minced parsley

1 In a large stockpot, over medium-high heat, heat the oil. Add the onion, garlic, and green pepper and sauté for 3–4 minutes. Sprinkle the flour and cumin over the onion mixture and cook 1 more minute.

2 Add the remaining ingredients except the parsley and bring to a boil. Lower the heat to simmer and cover, and cook for 30–35 minutes.

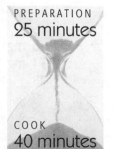

PREPARATION
25 minutes

COOK
40 minutes

Exchanges
2 Starch
1 Very Lean Meat

Calories 197
   Calories from Fat 25
Total Fat . . . . .3 g
   Saturated Fat . . . . .0 g
Cholesterol . . . . .0 mg
Sodium . . . . .204 mg
Carbohydrate . . . . .34 g
   Dietary Fiber . . . . .7 g
   Sugars . . . . 5 g
Protein . . . . .11 g

Red Bean Creole

Serving Size: 1/2 cup rice, 1 ounce sausage, Total Servings: 4

You can just picture cowboy legends sitting around their campfire preparing something similar to this. Our version is a bit more modern, but nonetheless still good grub!

2 tsp olive oil

2 cloves garlic, minced

1 cup diced onion

1/2 cup sliced celery

1/2 tsp chili powder

Salt and pepper to taste

2 cups fat-free, reduced-sodium chicken broth

1 cup long-grain rice

4 oz reduced-fat turkey sausage

1 cup canned red kidney beans, rinsed and drained

A few drops of hot pepper sauce

1 In a large skillet over medium-high heat, heat the oil. Add the garlic, onions, and celery and sauté for 4 minutes. Add the chili powder, salt, and pepper and sauté for 30 seconds. Add the broth and bring to a boil. Add the rice, bring to a second boil, lower the heat, cover, and simmer for 20 minutes.

2 Meanwhile, place the sausages in a saucepan covered with water. Bring to a boil. Lower the heat and simmer for 10–15 minutes until sausages are cooked through. Drain and allow to cool. Remove casings from the sausage and slice.

3 When the rice is done, add the sausage, kidney beans, and hot pepper sauce.

PREPARATION
15 minutes

COOK
35 minutes

Exchanges
3 1/2 Starch
1 Very Lean Meat

Calories 314
   Calories from Fat 36
Total Fat . . . . 4 g
   Saturated Fat . . . . .1 g
Cholesterol . . . . 12 mg
Sodium . . . . 577 mg
Carbohydrate . . . . 55 g
   Dietary Fiber . . . . 5 g
   Sugars . . . . 6 g
Protein . . . . .13 g

Tex-Mex Beans

Serving Size: about 1/2 cup, Total Servings: 4

Try Tex-Mex Beans topped with zesty salsa, all rolled inside a warm tortilla. Mash the beans slightly with a potato masher when you add them to the pan. This will make it easier to roll up the tortilla.

2 tsp olive oil	**1/2** tsp cumin
1/2 cup diced onion	**1** tsp mild chili powder
2 cloves garlic, minced	**2** cups red kidney beans
1 cup diced red pepper	**1** cup diced canned tomatoes, drained
1 tsp dried oregano	**1/2** cup shredded Monterey Jack cheese

1 In a skillet over medium-high heat, heat the oil. Add the onion, garlic, and peppers and sauté for 5 minutes. Add the oregano, cumin, and chili powder and sauté for 1 minute.

2 Add the beans and tomatoes and lower the heat. Simmer for 5 minutes.

3 Add the cheese, cover the skillet for 1–2 minutes until cheese melts.

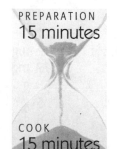

PREPARATION
15 minutes

COOK
15 minutes

Exchanges
1 1/2 Starch
1 Medium-fat Meat
1 Vegetable

Calories 217
    Calories from Fat 63
Total Fat . . . . 7 g
    Saturated Fat . . . . 3 g
Cholesterol . . . . 12 mg
Sodium . . . . 211 mg
Carbohydrate . . . . 28 g
    Dietary Fiber . . . . 8 g
    Sugars . . . . 7 g
Protein . . . . 12 g

Shrimp and Bean Skillet

Serving Size: about 4 ounces, Total Servings: 4

Think of this dish as a last-minute put-together. Just stop on your way home to pick up fresh shrimp. Everything else you probably have on hand.

2 tsp olive oil

1/2 cup diced onion

1 cup diced red pepper

1/2 cup diced celery

1 pound peeled and deveined medium shrimp

1 cup canned black-eyed peas or black beans, rinsed and drained

2 Tbsp minced parsley

Salt and pepper to taste

Dash crushed red pepper

1 In a medium skillet over medium-high heat, heat the oil. Add the onion and sauté for 2 minutes. Add the red pepper and sauté for 2 minutes. Add the celery and sauté for 2 minutes.

2 Add the shrimp and sauté until the shrimp turn pink about 5–6 minutes. Add the beans and parsley. Season with salt, pepper, and crushed red pepper. Cook 1 more minute.

PREPARATION
15 minutes

COOK
15 minutes

Exchanges
1/2 Starch
3 Very Lean Meat
1 Vegetable

Calories 171
  Calories from Fat 29
Total Fat . . . . .3 g
  Saturated Fat . . . . .0 g
Cholesterol . . . . .161 mg
Sodium . . . . 269 mg
Carbohydrate . . . . .14 g
  Dietary Fiber . . . . 4 g
  Sugars . . . . 4 g
Protein . . . . .21 g

Herbed Chickpeas and Potatoes

Serving Size: about 3/4 cup, Total Servings: 4

The combination of chickpeas and potatoes is an Indian tradition. Here we've used a bit more of the American flavors. The beans and potatoes are very filling. All you need is a green salad on the side.

2 medium russet potatoes, peeled and cubed into 1/2-inch cubes	**2** Tbsp minced parsley
2 tsp olive oil	**2** tsp minced oregano
1 cup diced carrots	**1** tsp minced thyme
1/2 cup diced onion	**1** tsp minced mint
2 cloves garlic, minced	**1 1/2** cups canned chickpeas, drained
2/3 cup diced canned tomatoes, drained	Salt and pepper to taste

1 Bring a saucepan filled with water to a boil. Add the potatoes and cook for 8–10 minutes until tender. Drain. Set aside.

2 In a skillet over medium-high heat, add the oil. Add the carrots and onions and sauté for 6–8 minutes. Add the garlic and sauté for 1 minute. Add the tomatoes and lower the heat to simmer. Add the parsley, oregano, thyme, and mint and simmer for 5 minutes.

3 Add the potatoes and chickpeas to the skillet and simmer for 2 minutes. Season with salt and pepper.

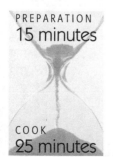

PREPARATION
15 minutes

COOK
25 minutes

Exchanges
2 Starch
1 Vegetable
1/2 Fat

Calories 199
 Calories from Fat 35
Total Fat . . . . 4 g
 Saturated Fat . . . . 0 g
Cholesterol . . . . 0 mg
Sodium . . . . 189 mg
Carbohydrate . . . . 35 g
 Dietary Fiber . . . . 8 g
 Sugars . . . . 9 g
Protein . . . . 8 g

Couscous Bean Pilaf

Serving Size: about 3/4 cup, Total Servings: 4

Serve with a broiled chicken breast or on its own as a main meal with a salad. Try it chilled the next day, piled high on a bed of crisp greens.

2 tsp olive oil
2 cloves garlic, minced
1/2 cup diced onion
1/2 cup diced carrot
1 Tbsp minced basil
1 cup dry couscous

1 1/2 cups fat-free, reduced-sodium chicken broth, heated
1 cup canned chickpeas, drained
1/4 cup toasted chopped walnuts
Salt and pepper to taste

1 In a skillet over medium-high heat, heat the oil. Add the garlic, onion, and carrot and sauté for 5 minutes. Add the basil and couscous and sauté for 1 minute.

2 Slowly add the hot broth to the pan, stir, cover, and remove from the heat. Let the couscous stand for 5–6 minutes until the liquid is absorbed.

3 Add the chickpeas and walnuts. Season with salt and pepper.

PREPARATION
15 minutes

COOK
6 minutes, 5–6 minutes standing time

Exchanges
3 1/2 Starch
1 Fat

Calories 320
   Calories from Fat 72
Total Fat . . . . 8 g
   Saturated Fat . . . . 0 g
Cholesterol . . . . 0 mg
Sodium . . . . 252 mg
Carbohydrate . . . . 51 g
   Dietary Fiber . . . . 7 g
   Sugars . . . . 6 g
Protein . . . . .12 g

Starchy Vegetables

Starchy vegetables, such as corn, peas, and all types of potatoes, are in the starch group because they have more carbohydrate than other, nonstarchy vegetables, such as broccoli, green beans, and tomatoes.

Don't steer away from starchy vegetables because of old-school beliefs about starchy vegetables and their effect on blood glucose. They don't raise blood glucose any more or quicker than other starches. And they've got some great nutrition assets, such as fiber, vitamins A and C, and potassium.

For most of the starchy vegetables, 1/2 cup is one serving or starch exchange. One serving has about 15 grams carbohydrate, 3 grams protein, 0-1 gram fat, and about 80 calories.

Sweet potatoes

Sweet potatoes are excellent sources of vitamins A and C, and good sources of vitamin B6 and copper.

How to Buy: Available all year long. Choose small- to medium-sized ones with smooth, unbruised skins. If the potato has "eyes," it's past its purchase time.

How to Store: Store in a cool, dry place and use within a week of purchase. Do not refrigerate them.

Uses: A sweet potato can be baked, boiled, roasted, or sautéed. Use to make potato salad, stews, soups, main dishes, side dishes, in baked goods, and desserts.

Sweet Potato Fries

Serving Size: 1 potato, Total Servings: 4

Our all-time favorite! This recipe is a hit even for those who think they dislike sweet potatoes. The familiarity of a "fry" really helps. A superb way to benefit from the sweet potato nutritional profile in a way everyone will enjoy.

4 small sweet potatoes, peel left on	Salt and pepper to taste
1 Tbsp olive oil	Cinnamon to taste

1 Preheat the oven to 450°F. Slice the potatoes lengthwise and then cut into 2-inch strips, ending up with about 20 slices per potato.

2 In a bowl, toss the potatoes with oil, salt, pepper, and cinnamon. Spread the potatoes in a single layer on a large baking sheet. Use two sheets if you need to.

3 Bake at 450°F for 25 minutes until soft and crunchy.

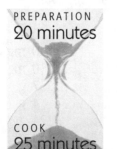

PREPARATION
20 minutes

COOK
25 minutes

Exchanges
1 1/2 Starch
1/2 Fat

Calories 130
   Calories from Fat 28
Total Fat . . . . .3 g
   Saturated Fat . . . . .1 g
Cholesterol . . . . .0 mg
Sodium . . . . .10 mg
Carbohydrate . . . . .24 g
   Dietary Fiber . . . . .3 g
   Sugars . . . . .11 g
Protein . . . . .2 g

Festive Sweet Potatoes

Serving Size: 1 potato, Total Servings: 4

Forget the gobs of butter and brown sugar. Pineapple and spices add the flavor, not the unwanted calories and fat.

4 sweet potatoes (3–4 oz each)

2 cups crushed pineapple, in its own juice

2 tsp cinnamon

1 tsp nutmeg

1 Tbsp slivered almonds (garnish)

1 To cook sweet potatoes, either boil, unpeeled, in a large pot and let them cook over medium heat for 45 minutes, uncovered, until you can put a fork in them easily. Or you can bake the sweet potatoes in a preheated 375°F oven directly on the rack for 45 minutes to 1 hour.

2 Preheat the oven to 350°F. Let the cooked potatoes cool and then gently peel them.

3 Mash the potatoes with the pineapple and spices. Put in a 1-quart casserole dish and top with slivered almonds. Bake for 20 minutes until potatoes are lightly browned.

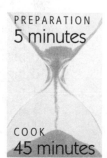

PREPARATION
5 minutes

COOK
45 minutes

Exchanges
1 1/2 Starch
1 Fruit

Calories 162
   Calories from Fat 11
Total Fat . . . . .1 g
   Saturated Fat . . . . .0 g
Cholesterol . . . . .0 mg
Sodium . . . . 10 mg
Carbohydrate . . . . .37 g
   Dietary Fiber . . . . .4 g
   Sugars . . . . 24 g
Protein . . . . .2 g

Avoid potatoes that have sprouted or have a wilted or wrinkled skin, cut surfaces, green or dark areas, or worm holes. Store them in a cool, dry, dark place that is well-ventilated. Don't wash them before storage. The ideal storage temperature is 40–50°F, but most potatoes will keep for two weeks at room temperature. Don't put potatoes in the refrigerator; some of the starch will be converted to sugar making them taste too sweet, and the potato will darken when cooked.

The **Yukon Gold** has a buttery, sweet flavor. Fine for baking, mashing, and roasting. Most grocery stores now carry this great spud, so do try it. Try them mashed first, you will find you need absolutely no butter!

Yellow Finns have a sweet taste and look similar to Yukons. Use them in any recipe calling for a russet.

The **Russet of Idaho** potato is the best-known and best-loved of all the potatoes. Available everywhere, the russet is an all-purpose potato. We think it is best for a classic baked potato. It's also the best potato for soup, because it holds its shape.

New potatoes are not really a separate variety but rather are young, small potatoes of any variety that are harvested in the first nine months of the year. Their skin is thin and wispy. They are wonderful served steamed or boiled.

Serve Them Up!

Skip the butter and sour cream and get creative with spuds!

- Make a "pizza" potato: Top a cooked spud with low-fat marinara sauce and 1-2 tsp Parmesan cheese. Place back in the oven until bubbly.
- Put a little zip into the potato by topping it with any bottled salsa (about 2 Tbsp per serving), canned low-fat vegetarian chili (about 2 Tbsp per serving), mango chutney (about 1 Tbsp per serving), or 2 Tbsp melted low-fat shredded cheese mixed with 1 Tbsp salsa.
- Sauté mushrooms and onions in a bit of olive oil and pile high on the potato.
- Make a full meal: Sauté small shrimp in a bit of olive oil and garlic; add basil, oregano, and pepper; stuff into a baked potato.

- When making mashed potatoes, instead of butter, substitute just a little bit of olive oil whipped with low-fat chicken broth and herbs of your choice.
- Cube either red potatoes or Yukons and toss with Dijon mustard, a little white wine, and herbs, and bake until tender.
- Want to get really great taste? Slice any potato lengthwise into 1/2-inch pieces, toss with a bit of olive oil, and grill them until crusty and tender. Use a vegetable basket if the slices will fall through the grill rack.

Foil-Roasted Herb Potatoes

Serving Size: about 1/2 cup, Total Servings: 4

We often cook in foil in our test kitchen. It's so easy and there's no clean-up. Roasting the potatoes in foil ensures a moist potato, and the herbs will have a chance to flavor the potato completely. When you open the packet, take a few moments to savor the heady aroma.

1 lb Yukon Gold potatoes, cubed

2 Tbsp olive oil

2 sprigs rosemary

2 sprigs oregano

2 sprigs thyme

Salt and pepper to taste

1 tsp paprika

1 Preheat the oven to 400°F. Tear four large sheets of foil.

2 Divide all ingredients among the four sheets of foil. Wrap up the potatoes, seal tightly. Put all packets on a baking sheet.

3 Roast the potatoes in the oven for 35 minutes.

4 Place one packet on each dinner plate and allow diners to open their packets.

PREPARATION
15 minutes

COOK
35 minutes

Exchanges
1 1/2 Starch
1 Fat

Calories 146
　　Calories from Fat 55
Total Fat . . . . 6 g
　　Saturated Fat . . . . .1 g
Cholesterol . . . . 0 mg
Sodium . . . . 9 mg
Carbohydrate . . . . 21 g
　　Dietary Fiber . . . . 2 g
　　Sugars . . . . 2 g
Protein . . . . 3 g

Creamy Mashed Potatoes

Serving Size: about 3/4 cup, Total Servings: 4

When we want a more country-mashed potato, we use a potato masher. When we want it smooth, we use our ricer. Russet potatoes, in our opinion, still make the best mashed potato, though Yukon Golds are good too.

2 lbs russet potatoes, peeled and cut into 2-inch pieces

2 Tbsp olive oil

3 Tbsp low-fat sour cream

1/2 cup heated fat-free, reduced-sodium chicken broth

Salt and pepper to taste

1 In a large saucepan filled with boiling water, boil the potatoes for 20 to 25 minutes until cooked through. Drain.

2 Put them back in the pot over low heat, and shake them a bit to dry them. Stir in the remaining ingredients and mash well.

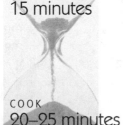

PREPARATION
15 minutes

COOK
20–25 minutes

Exchanges
2 1/2 Starch
1/2 Fat

Calories 220
    Calories from Fat 65
Total Fat . . . . 7 g
    Saturated Fat . . . . 2 g
Cholesterol . . . . 4 mg
Sodium . . . . 76 mg
Carbohydrate . . . . 36 g
    Dietary Fiber . . . . 3 g
    Sugars . . . . 3 g
Protein . . . . 4 g

Twice-Baked Potatoes

Serving Size: 1 potato, Total Servings: 4

This stuffed potato is so simple to prepare you won't ever bother with those high-fat frozen versions.

4 russet potatoes (about 8 oz each), scrubbed	**2** cloves garlic, minced
1/2 cup 1% milk, warmed	**1/2** tsp basil
1/4 cup Parmesan cheese	**1/4** tsp oregano
	Salt and pepper

1 Preheat the oven to 350°F. Bake the potatoes directly on the rack for about 1 hour until cooked through. Remove potatoes from the oven and let cool for about 15 minutes.

2 Split the potatoes in half lengthwise and scoop out the flesh. Combine the flesh with the remaining ingredients and stuff into potato shells.

3 Put potatoes on a baking sheet and bake at 350°F for 15 minutes.

PREPARATION
10 minutes

COOK
1 hour and 15 minutes

Exchanges
3 Starch

Calories 246
   Calories from Fat 25
Total Fat . . . . 3 g
   Saturated Fat . . . . 2 g
Cholesterol . . . . 9 mg
Sodium . . . . .156 mg
Carbohydrate . . . . 48 g
   Dietary Fiber . . . . 4 g
   Sugars . . . . 5 g
Protein . . . . 9 g

DELICIOUS TOPPINGS FOR BAKED POTATOES, RICE, AND PASTA

Use any of the following toppings for 1 baked potato, or 1 cup cooked pasta or rice. Use a medium-sized skillet for all recipes. Makes 1 serving.

Italiano

Sauté 1/4 cup of minced onion in 1/2 tsp olive oil over medium-high heat. Add 1 tsp minced garlic and sauté 1 minute. Add 1/2 cup canned diced tomatoes, 2 tsp tomato paste, 1/2 tsp dried basil, and 1/4 tsp dried oregano. Add 2 tsp red or white wine if desired. Bring to a boil, lower the heat, and simmer for 5 minutes.

Asian vegetable

Sauté 1 tsp minced ginger and 1/2 tsp minced garlic in 1/2 tsp peanut oil for 1 minute. Add 1/4 cup diced red pepper, 1/4 cup broccoli florets, and 1/4 cup sliced carrot. Stir-fry for 3 minutes. Add 1/4 cup fat-free, reduced-sodium chicken broth, cover, and steam for 2-3 minutes. Add 1 Tbsp light soy sauce.

Mexicali

Sauté 1/4 cup diced onion and 1 tsp minced garlic in 1/2 tsp canola oil for 2 minutes. Add 1 small tomato, seeded and diced, and 2 Tbsp corn and sauté for 2 minutes. Add in 1/4 tsp chili powder and 2 tsp minced cilantro.

French

Sauté 1/4 cup diced onion and 1 tsp minced garlic in 1/2 tsp hazelnut, walnut, or olive oil for 2-3 minutes. Add in 1/2 cup trimmed green beans, 1/2 tsp dried thyme, 1 Tbsp chopped black olives, and 1/4 cup fat-free, reduced-sodium chicken broth. Cover and steam for 2-3 minutes until green beans are crisp and bright green.

Greek

Sauté 1/4 cup diced red onion and 1 tsp minced garlic in 1/2 tsp olive oil for 2-3 minutes. Add in 1/4 cup sliced white mushrooms and sauté for 3 minutes. Add 1/2 cup tomatoes, seeded and diced, and sauté for 2 minutes. Add 1/2 tsp dried thyme and 1/4 tsp dried oregano and 1 tsp lemon juice and cook for 1 minute. Add 2 tsp crumbled feta cheese.

CORN

Despite its reputation for being fattening, a 3-inch ear of corn has only 80 calories and is low in fat.

Selecting Corn

Corn is so much better in summer, so buy it then. To select a good ear of corn, pull back the husk and look at the kernels. They should look plump, juicy, and full-colored. Avoid corn with kernels spaced far apart or that look dry.

Cooking Corn

In a pot: Fill a large stockpot with 6 quarts of water. Peel off the husks and silks of the corn. Bring the water to a boil. Add the corn. Bring to another boil. Cover the pot, turn off the heat, and let stand for 5 minutes. Drain.

Grilling: Peel back the husks and remove the silks. Replace the husks back over the corn and tie the ends with twine to secure. Soak the ears in salted water for 15 minutes. (Salt water helps keep the husks from burning.) Place the husks on the grill for 10-15 minutes over medium heat until kernels are bright yellow.

In the microwave: Wrap the husks in wet paper towels. Cook 4 minutes on high.

In the oven: Preheat the oven to 425ºF. Prepare the corn as for grilling. Roast the corn for 20 minutes on the rack until the kernels are bright yellow.

Chive Corn Pudding

Serving Size: about 1 cup, Total Servings: 4

When Robyn was in graduate school in the South, corn pudding was a staple on the menu. Here we've lightened it up a little by using low-fat milk, low-fat sour cream, and reduced-fat cheese.

2 ears corn, husks and silks removed; or 2 cups frozen corn, thawed

2 cups 1% milk

2 Tbsp low-fat sour cream

2 eggs

2 Tbsp flour

1 Tbsp sugar

2 Tbsp minced chives

1/2 cup low-fat cheddar cheese

1 Preheat the oven to 350°F. If using fresh corn, use a sharp knife to scrape the corn from the cob.

2 Combine the corn with the remaining ingredients in a food processor or blender.

3 Spray a casserole dish with nonstick spray. Pour the corn pudding into the casserole dish.

4 Bake uncovered for 35–40 minutes until pudding is set and tester put in the center comes out clean.

PREPARATION
10 minutes

COOK
40 minutes

Exchanges
1 1/2 Starch   1 Lean Meat
1/2 Fat-free Milk
(Or 2 Carbohydrate + 1 Lean Meat)

Calories 215
    Calories from Fat 52
Total Fat . . . . 6 g
    Saturated Fat . . . . 3 g
Cholesterol . . . . .115 mg
Sodium . . . . .196 mg
Carbohydrate . . . . 29 g
    Dietary Fiber . . . . 2 g
    Sugars . . . . .10 g
Protein . . . . .14 g

Vegetable Burritos

Serving Size: 1 tortilla, Total Servings: 4

You can make a burrito without all the fat-laden cheese. This burrito is chock-full of ingredients that are high in fiber and taste. Although white-flour tortillas are not the worst, try to get a whole-wheat tortilla. We think the whole-wheat tastes better. Whole-wheat tortillas are available at gourmet stores, some health food stores, and some major supermarkets.

4 whole-wheat tortillas (medium: 7–8″)

1 Tbsp olive oil

2 cloves garlic, minced

1 yellow onion, minced

1 red pepper, diced

1 cup yellow corn, cooked (off the cob or frozen)

1 cup canned black beans (rinsed and drained), mashed slightly (use a potato masher)

1 Tbsp chili powder

2 tsp cumin

1 tsp chopped cilantro

Your favorite salsa

1 Warm the tortillas in one of three ways: Wrap the tortillas in foil and warm them in a 300°F oven. Or warm them one at a time by drying in a skillet on each side for 1 minute and then keep them warm until assembly time. Or put the tortillas in a stack with a paper towel between each tortilla. Set the stack in the microwave and microwave on high for about 30 seconds.

2 To prepare the filling: Heat the oil in a large skillet or wok. Add the garlic, onions, and red pepper and sauté for 2 minutes. Add the corn and beans and cook another 2 minutes. Add the chili powder, cumin, and cilantro. Cook an additional 1 minute.

3 To assemble: Spoon some of the bean-corn mixture on one end of each tortilla. Fold in the two sides of the tortilla and then carefully roll the tortilla to encase the filling. Repeat with each tortilla. Serve with salsa.

PREPARATION
20 minutes

COOK
5 minutes

Exchanges

3 Starch   1 Vegetable
1 Fat

Calories 308
    Calories from Fat 67
Total Fat . . . . .7 g
    Saturated Fat . . . . .2 g
Cholesterol . . . . .0 mg
Sodium . . . . .313 mg
Carbohydrate . . . . .53 g
    Dietary Fiber . . . . .9 g
    Sugars . . . . .7 g
Protein . . . . .10 g

Glazed Parsnips

Serving Size: about 1/2 cup, Total Servings: 8

Parsnips are root vegetables. Fresh parsnips are pleasantly sweet and really good roasted.

Choose young, straight, firm roots without blemish. Avoid large roots, as they tend to be woody. Parsnips can be stored unwashed in a perforated bag in the refrigerator for one week.

People often just boil and mash parsnips as they would potatoes, but we think parsnips deserve a little more imagination. Parsnips are also suitable for almost any other method of cooking.

1 lb parsnips

2 Tbsp olive oil, divided

2 Tbsp brown sugar

Salt and pepper to taste

1 Preheat the oven to 400°F. Trim both ends of the parsnips and peel. Cut the parsnips in half lengthwise, then slice into matchstick strips.

2 In a medium bowl, toss the parsnips with 1 Tbsp of the olive oil. Spread the parsnips on a baking sheet in a single layer. Roast the parsnips for 15 minutes.

3 In a small bowl, combine the remaining oil, brown sugar, and salt and pepper to taste. Sprinkle over the parsnips and continue to bake for 15 more minutes until parsnips are cooked through and slightly crispy.

PREPARATION
20 minutes

COOK
30 minutes

Exchanges
1 Starch

Calories 79
Calories from Fat 28
Total Fat . . . . 3 g
Saturated Fat . . . . 1 g
Cholesterol . . . . 0 mg
Sodium . . . . 6 mg
Carbohydrate . . . . .13 g
Dietary Fiber . . . . 2 g
Sugars . . . . 5 g
Protein . . . . .1 g

Butternut Squash and Pear Soup

Serving Size: about 1 cup, Total Servings: 6

If we were to pick one of our favorite soups of all time, this would be it. You will see butternut squash recipes calling for the squash to be boiled. We prefer to roast the squash, which enhances the flavor. The pears give this soup definite fall feel.

1 medium (about 1 lb) butternut squash

2 medium Bartlett or D'Anjou pears

1 medium onion, sliced vertically

1 clove garlic, minced

2 Tbsp butter

2 cups fat-free, reduced-sodium chicken broth

1 1/2 cups evaporated skim milk

Salt and pepper to taste

1 Preheat the oven to 400°F. Cut the squash in half, scoop out the seeds, and discard the seeds. If you have trouble cutting through the squash, place the squash, whole, in the microwave and microwave for 5-6 minutes. Remove from the microwave. It should now be easier to cut through the squash.

2 Remove the stem from each pear and cut each pear in half and scoop out the core.

3 In a casserole dish large enough to accommodate the squash, place the sliced onion, garlic, and butter on the bottom. Top with the squash halves and pear halves, cut side down. Roast for 30–45 minutes until squash is cooked through and pears are soft.

4 Scoop the flesh out of the squash and puree in a blender with the rest of the contents of the casserole dish.

5 In a large saucepan over medium heat, heat the broth. Add the puree and cook for 5–6 minutes. Lower the heat to simmer and simmer for 10 minutes. Add the milk and simmer for 5 minutes. Season with salt and pepper.

PREPARATION
20 minutes

COOK
1 hour

Exchanges
1 1/2 Carbohydrate
1 Fat

Calories 152
   Calories from Fat 41
Total Fat . . . . .5 g
   Saturated Fat . . . . .2 g
Cholesterol . . . . .10 mg
Sodium . . . . 282 mg
Carbohydrate . . . . .22 g
   Dietary Fiber . . . . .3 g
   Sugars . . . . 16 g
Protein . . . . .7 g

SECTION

4 Grains, Beans, and Starchy Vegetables

	Exchange/ Serving	Calories	Carbohydrate (g)	Protein (g)	Fat (g)	Fiber (g)
GRAINS						
Breads						
Bagel	1/2 (35 g)	98	19	4	0.5	1
Bread, pumpernickel	1 slice	80	15	3	1	2
Bread, rye	1 slice	83	16	3	1	2
Bread, white, reduced-calorie	2 slices	96	20	4	1	4
Bread, white, French, Italian	1 slice	67	12	2	1	1
Bread, whole-wheat	1 slice	70	13	3	1	2
Bread sticks	2	82	14	2	2	1
English muffin	1/2	67	13	2	0.5	1
Hamburger bun	1/2	61	11	2	1	1
Hot dog bun	1/2	61	11	2	1	1
Pita bread (6" dia.)	1/2	83	17	3	0.5	1
Raisin bread	1 slice	71	14	2	1	1
Roll, plain	1	85	14	2	2	1
Tortilla, corn, 6–7"	1	56	12	1	0.5	1
Tortilla, flour, 7–8"	1	114	20	3	2.5	1
Waffle, reduced-fat, 4 1/2" square	1	80	16	2	0.5	1
Cereals, cold						
All Bran	1/2 cup	75	22	4	1	10
Bran Buds	1/2 cup	112	33	6	1	16
Cheerios	3/4 cup	90	16	4	0	2
Cornflakes	3/4 cup	89	20	2	0	1
Granola, low-fat	1/2 cup	105	21	2	1.5	2
Grape nuts	1/4 cup	105	24	4	0	2
Grapenut flakes	3/4 cup	104	24	3	0	3
Kix	3/4 cup	66	14	2	0	0
Product 19	3/4 cup	88	20	2	0	1
Puffed rice	1 1/2 cups	90	22	2	0	0
Puffed wheat	1 1/2 cups	76	15	3	0	1

(continued)

Grains, Beans, and Starchy Vegetables

	Exchange/ Serving	Calories	Carbohydrate (g)	Protein (g)	Fat (g)	Fiber (g)
Cereals, cold (cont'd)						
Raisin bran	1/2 cup	85	22	2	0.5	4
Rice Krispies	3/4 cup	71	16	1	0	0
Shredded wheat	1/2 cup	90	20	3	0.5	2
Sugar frosted flakes	1/2 cup	67	16	1	0	0
Wheaties	3/4 cup	80	18	2	0	2
Cereals, cooked						
Cream of rice	1/2 cup	63	14	1	0	0
Cream of wheat	1/2 cup	67	14	2	0	1
Grits	1/2 cup	73	16	2	0	0
Oatmeal	1/2 cup	73	13	3	1	2
Whole wheat	1/2 cup	75	17	2	0.5	2
Crackers and Snacks						
Animal crackers	8	89	15	1	3	0
Crispbread	2 slices	73	16	2	0.5	3
Graham crackers	3	89	16	1	2	1
Matzos	3/4 oz	83	18	2	0.5	1
Melba toast	4 slices	78	15	2	0.5	1
Oyster crackers	24	78	13	2	2	0
Popcorn, popped, no fat added	3 cups	92	19	3	1	4
Popcorn, microwave, light (1/2 bag)	3 cups	65	11	2	2	2
Pretzels, sticks/rings	3/4 oz	80	17	2	1	1
Rice cake, regular	2	70	15	2	0.5	1
Rye crisp	3 slices	86	20	2	0	2
Tortilla chips, not fried	17	82	18	2	1	3
Triscuits, reduced fat	5 wafers	81	15	2	2	2
Grains						
Bulgur, cooked	1/2 cup	76	17	3	0	4
Cornmeal, dry, degermed	3 Tbsp	97	20	2	0.5	2
Couscous, cooked	1/3 cup	67	14	2	0	1
Flour, white	3 Tbsp	87	18	2	0	1

(continued)

Grains, Beans, and Starchy Vegetables

	Exchange/ Serving	Calories	Carbohydrate (g)	Protein (g)	Fat (g)	Fiber (g)
Kasha	1/2 cup	91	20	3	1	2
Millet, cooked	1/4 cup	72	14	2	1	1
Rice, white, long grain, cooked	1/3 cup	69	15	1	0	0
Rice, brown, cooked	1/3 cup	72	15	2	1	1
Wheat germ, toasted	3 Tbsp	80	10	6	2	3
Pasta						
Macaroni, cooked firm	1/2 cup	99	20	3	0.5	1
Noodles, enriched egg, cooked	1/2 cup	106	20	4	1	1
Spaghetti, cooked firm	1/2 cup	99	20	3	0.5	1

BEANS, PEAS, LENTILS (Count as 1 starch and 1 very lean meat exchange)

	Exchange/ Serving	Calories	Carbohydrate (g)	Protein (g)	Fat (g)	Fiber (g)
Beans						
Baked	1/3 cup	79	17	4	0.5	4
Garbanzo (chickpeas), cooked	1/2 cup	134	22	7	2	4
Kidney, canned	1/2 cup	105	19	7	0.5	4
Kidney, cooked	1/2 cup	112	20	8	0.5	6
Lima	2/3 cup	114	21	7	0.5	8
Lima, canned	2/3 cup	125	23	8	0.5	5
Navy, cooked	1/2 cup	129	24	8	0.5	6
Pinto, cooked	1/2 cup	117	22	7	0.5	7
White, cooked	1/2 cup	126	23	9	0.5	6
Peas, split, cooked	1/2 cup	117	21	8	0.5	8
Peas, black-eyed, cooked	1/2 cup	100	18	7	0.5	6
Lentils, cooked	1/2 cup	117	20	9	0.5	8
Miso (sodium)	3 Tbsp	106	14	6	3	3

STARCHY VEGETABLES

	Exchange/ Serving	Calories	Carbohydrate (g)	Protein (g)	Fat (g)	Fiber (g)
Corn, frozen, cooked	1/2 cup	66	17	2	0	2
Corn, whole kernel, vac. pack	1/2 cup	83	20	2	0.5	2

(continued)

Grains, Beans, and Starchy Vegetables

	Exchange/ Serving	Calories	Carbohydrate (g)	Protein (g)	Fat (g)	Fiber (g)
STARCHY VEGETABLES (cont'd)						
Corn on cob, cooked, medium (5 oz)	1 cob	83	19	3	1	2
Corn on cob, frozen, 3"	1 cob	70	14	2	0.5	1
Mixed vegetables with corn	1 cup	80	18	4	0	4
Mixed vegetables with pasta	1 cup	80	15	3	0	5
Peas, green, canned, drained	1/2 cup	59	11	4	0.5	4
Peas, green, frozen, cooked	1/2 cup	62	11	4	0	4
Plantain, cooked slices	1/2 cup	89	24	1	0	2
Potato, baked with skin	3 oz	93	22	2	0	2
Potato, white, peeled, boiled	3 oz	73	17	2	0	2
Potato, mashed, flakes (with milk and fat)	1/2 cup	119	16	2	6	2
Squash, winter	1 cup	83	22	2	0	7
Potato, sweet, canned, vac. pack, pieces	1/2 cup	92	22	2	0	3
Yam, plain	1/2 cup	79	19	1	0	2

(sodium) = 400 mg or more of sodium per exchange.

FOCUS ON Portion Control

"I don't understand why I'm not losing weight. I'm eating all the right foods."

"I'm following my meal plan, but my blood sugars are higher than I expected. Why?"

Have you ever found yourself with these questions? If the answer you came up with is "I'm just eating too much of the right foods," you've hit the nail on the head. Yes, choosing the right types of foods to eat is important, but it's just as important to eat the right amounts of those foods. It's not just what you eat, it's how much you eat, too!

Surprisingly, the extra calories from portions that are just a bit too large add up quickly. Perhaps it's an extra quarter-cup of cereal at breakfast, an extra ounce of turkey in a sandwich with a larger-than-medium apple at lunch, and an extra half-cup of pasta, another ounce of steak, and an extra tablespoon of salad dressing at dinner.

It's easy to rationalize these "extras" as nothing that will prevent you from achieving your diabetes and nutrition goals. After all, it's not a candy bar or slice of cheesecake! True, but these "extras" on a daily basis can mean you gain 2 pounds rather than lose 2 pounds, or that you don't meet your blood glucose goals.

To keep on track with portions, put the tools and tricks of the trade to work.

Tools for Portion Control

Open your cabinets and you will likely find a few of the portion control essentials: measuring spoons, and liquid and solid measuring cups. Rather than keeping them in the deep, dark trenches of your cabinets, find them a new, easy-to-grab location in your kitchen: a corner of the counter or a within-reach cabinet. You want your measuring tools to beg to be used.

Measuring spoons

Have a set of measuring spoons with at least 1/2 and 1 teaspoon, and 1 tablespoon. There are 3 teaspoons in 1 tablespoon. Don't rely on your teaspoons and tablespoons from your table-service set. They vary in size based on style and aren't an exact measure.

Measuring cup for liquids

Have a 1-cup liquid measuring cup. A liquid measuring cup should be clear (glass or clear plastic) so you can see through it. To measure liquids correctly, get down at eye level to make sure the liquid reaches the right line.

Measuring cups for solids

Have a set of 1/4 cup, 1/2 cup, 3/4 cup, and 1 cup. Use the size cup equal to the portion you want to measure and fill it to the top. Level it with the flat edge of a knife to eliminate any excess.

Food scale

Get at least an inexpensive ($5–$10) food scale, particularly for measuring foods you measure in ounces, such as meat, fish, or cheese.

More expensive scales are available, but they aren't necessary. You can spend a low of $25 to a high of $190. On the low end, the food scale gives ounces, pounds, grams, and kilograms and is more precise than the lower-cost variety. On the high end, there are digital scales that give you an exact measure to read rather than reading between the lines.

Eyeballs

Don't underestimate a pair of well-trained and honest eyeballs. They are an invaluable measuring tool because they are always at the ready— at home, in restaurants, or at the soccer field.

Nutrition Facts on the food label

The Nutrition Facts label you find on most packaged foods today is one of your best portion control aids because it must list the serving size. That can help you learn what reasonable portions are. If you usually eat a larger quantity of that food, perhaps your portions are too large or the portion you eat should count as 2 servings. But keep in mind that the food label serving size is not always the same as the diabetes serving or exchange (see p. 299).

Tricks of the Trade

Weigh and measure your foods often when you get started or when you eat a food that is difficult for you to guestimate the portion.

Always serve in the same size plates, glasses, and bowls. This helps you judge correct portions and decreases how often you need to use measuring tools. For example, use the same glass for milk. Once or twice, measure your milk out in a measuring cup and pour it into the glass. See where that quantity comes to. You may want to mark it with an indelible marker. See how much room one cup of pasta takes on a dinner plate, one-half cup of hot oatmeal in a bowl, and so on. Keep these pictures in your mind.

When you feel confident that you can eyeball correctly, don't feel you have to weigh and measure everything. Just do so from time to time, perhaps once a week, just to make sure your eyeballs don't grow with time.

Quiz yourself occasionally. Measure cereal, pasta, or rice in the container you eat it in. Then measure the quantity you poured. For example, pour your milk from your glass into a measuring cup. Are your portions correct? If not, readjust your eyeballs with measuring equipment.

HANDY HAND GUIDES

Here are some handy hand guides to help you guestimate portions. Use these when you eat in restaurants, at a friend or relative's house, or as a check when you eat at home and feel you have mastered weighing and measuring your foods.

Thumb tip = 1 teaspoon
Example: 1 teaspoon of mayonnaise, salad dressing, or margarine

Thumb = 1 ounce
Example: 1 ounce of cheese or meat

Palm = 3 ounces
Example: 3 ounces of cooked meat (with no bone)

Tight fist = 1/2 cup
Example: 1 serving of pasta, 1 serving of canned fruit

Handful = 1 cup
Example: 2 servings of pasta, 2 servings cooked vegetable

RECIPES

VEGETABLES

3 Flavored Vinegars ———————————— 100

5 Easy Dressings with Low-fat Sour Cream ———— 101

✈ Roasted Garlic ———————————— 103

✈ Caramelized Onions ———————————— 104

✈ Green Beans with Tomatoes and Herbs —— 105

✈ Zucchini Marinara ———————————— 106

✈ Broccoli with Sesame Seeds
and Scallions ———————————— 108

✈ Broccoli and Garlic ———————————— 109

✈ Brussels Sprouts with Chestnuts ———— 110

✈ Cauliflower with Cheddar Cheese Sauce —— 111

✈ Curried Cauliflower Soup ———————— 112

✈ Healthy Coleslaw ———————————— 113

✈ Fall Spinach Salad ———————————— 114

✈ Soy Kale ———————————————— 115

✈ Arugula and Watercress Salad ————— 116

✈ Spinach Sauté with Mushrooms ———— 117

The message you hear broadcast over and over is **eat more vegetables**. The more nutrition experts learn about foods and health, the better vegetables look.

Vegetables are packed with vitamins and minerals and have few calories. They have fiber. They have no fat, no saturated fat, and no cholesterol—in their unadulterated state. Sure, you can easily pack calories and fat into vegetables without trying too hard. Consider spinach soufflé, broccoli with cheese sauce, or a salad with several heaping tablespoons of blue cheese dressing. As usual, nutritious preparation of vegetables is key. Keep the fat low and preserve nutrients with minimal cooking.

On average, 1 vegetable serving or exchange contains about 5 grams of carbohydrate, 2 grams of protein, and 25 calories.

The diabetes food pyramid suggests you eat 3 to 5 servings of vegetables each day. One serving, or 1 vegetable exchange, is usually 1/2 cup cooked vegetables, 1/2 cup vegetable juice, or 1 cup raw vegetables.

EAT THE RAINBOW OF VEGETABLES

While all vegetables are good sources of vitamins and minerals, variety is definitely the spice of life because different vegetables offer you their various strong suits. Keep the colors green, yellow, and red in mind when you choose your vegetables.

- Dark-green, leafy vegetables (Nutrition Superstars) are good sources of beta carotene, which forms vitamin A. Other green vegetables, such as broccoli, green peppers, and Brussels sprouts, are good sources of vitamin C.
- Deep yellow vegetables, such as carrots and butternut squash, are good sources of beta carotene.
- Deep red vegetables, such as tomatoes and red peppers, are good sources of vitamin C.

In addition, vegetables contain phytochemicals, a diverse group of natural substances found in plants. (Phyto comes from the Greek word for plant.) Some of the ones you may have heard of are carotenoids, isoflavones, and protease inhibitors.

Phytochemicals may offer some protection against certain types of cancer and heart disease.

Fruits and vegetables contain hundreds of phytochemicals, and it's suspected that they contain many more that are as yet unknown.

Antioxidants

Antioxidants are a group of phytochemicals that have been getting a lot of publicity.

When the body's cells burn oxygen, molecules called free radicals form. It's thought that free radicals damage the body's cells. This "oxidative stress" may play a role in the development of cancer, heart disease, cataracts, and the aging process.

Antioxidants seem to combat the effects of free radicals by neutralizing them. The antioxidants most often mentioned are beta carotene, vitamin C, vitamin E, and selenium. Carotenoids other than beta carotene that are becoming better known are alpha carotene, lycopene, lutein, and zeaxanthin.

It's thought that high blood glucose levels may contribute to oxidative stress. According to the American Diabetes Association, more research is needed before a recommendation about antioxidant supplementation for people with diabetes. Eating a wide variety of fruits and vegetables every day is the best protection.

SHOPPING FOR PRODUCE

Perhaps no other department in the market will give you the variety and abundance of nutrition than the produce department. The dizzying array of selections can confuse anyone. Here is what you need to be a savvy consumer.

First and foremost, give the entire section a once-over. Check to see that the produce looks fresh, that there are water sprayers for lettuces and greens, and that in general the section looks clean and well organized.

Break out of your ruts! Add a new fruit or vegetable to your cart once every other week. The key to a well balanced eating plan is variety. Ask the produce manager for tips on how to use the fruit or vegetable.

Look for quality. Avoid any fruit or vegetable that is bruised or looks old. There is often a separate shelf in the market labeled: "Reduced for Quick Sale." Although it may be appealing to purchase really inexpensive produce, the nutritional value of these foods may be low.

Most vegetables will not come with nutritional labeling, but oftentimes this information is available. Many markets now post that information in the form of posters and pamphlets available right in the produce department.

Don't get too carried away with eating healthy. This may sound funny, but don't purchase a truckload of perishable fruits and vegetables only to throw half of it out. Use your weekly planner as a guide.

If you are finding you are throwing out more produce than you are eating, consider buying frozen and canned versions. Choose frozen vegetables that are plain, not dressed with cream or cheese sauces. If possible, buy vegetables in bags versus boxes. It is much easier to seal up whatever you don't use.

Try to use up frozen vegetables in 3 to 4 months. Rotate the vegetables every time you purchase more. Place older vegetables up front and new ones in the back.

Fresh, Frozen, or Canned?

People often wonder whether canned and frozen vegetables are as good as fresh.

Vegetables vary in their nutrition depending on the soil they are grown in, the time of year they are grown, their ripeness when they are picked, and the length of time between when they are picked and when they are eaten, frozen, or canned. The nutrition that remains after cooking depends on the length of cooking time and the amount of liquid the vegetables are cooked in.

A vegetable picked at its peak and frozen very soon after will retain more nutrients than the same vegetable that is transported to your grocery store and then sits for several days before you buy it "fresh."

To get the most out of fresh vegetables: Buy locally-grown, in-season produce when you can. Buy the freshest-looking vegetables and eat them soon after. Try eating more of your vegetables raw.

Cook fresh or frozen vegetables in a very small amount of water for a short time to preserve nutrients. Look for canned vegetables with no added salt.

TIPS FOR EATING MORE VEGGIES

In the end, the best vegetables are the ones you eat. Buy what's most convenient. Here are easy ways to add vegetables (and their bounty of vitamins and minerals) to your diet:

- Remember there's always room for vegetables. When preparing a main dish, add a few vegetables. Preparing a tomato sauce for pasta or lasagna? Add sautéed onions, peppers, mushrooms, zucchini, or eggplant. Making a stuffing? Add shredded carrots, onions, and mushrooms. Enrich simple macaroni and cheese by adding some tomatoes, red peppers, and onion.
- If you hate to cut up vegetables or just feel you don't have time, take advantage of the supermarket offerings of pre-cut vegetables, packaged lettuces, and ready-to-fix salad bar. You'll be eating vegetables and still spending less than if you ate a restaurant meal.
- Let vegetables help you reduce protein. Making a meat loaf or meatballs? Add onions, carrots, peppers. Preparing an omelette? Add onions, tomatoes, peppers, mushrooms. Whipping up some tuna salad? Chop in some onions and carrots.
- Don't have a meat-only sandwich. Top it off with sprouts, onions, sliced peppers, cucumbers, tomatoes, or lettuce.
- Keep a bag of those little carrots around. Use them for a quick salad topper, a crunch along with a sandwich, or a dipper with a low-fat dressing.
- Stock your cupboard or freezer with canned or frozen vegetables. They'll be there at-the-ready for months, and they won't go brown.
- Consider cooking up 3 to 4 servings of a vegetable at one time. For example, cook a head of broccoli and cut it into bite-size pieces. Store it in a plastic container. Then it's ready for a quick vegetable at dinner, a topper for salad, a quick vegetable to dip for a snack. Cooked vegetables keep 1–2 days in the refrigerator.

THE SALAD BAR

Salads can be healthy . . . and not so healthy. Stay away from iceberg lettuce topped with egg, cheese, and gobs of high-fat dressing. Here are tips for healthy salads:

The Salad

- Add darker greens to salads, because the darker greens offer more nutrition. Give arugula, spinach, watercress, and romaine a try. Use them on sandwiches as well.

- One reason people don't eat salads is they hate to do all the tearing up. Here's one solution. Tear a bunch up at once and store in a plastic container. Grab a handful and you've got instant salad. Or buy a bag of pre-cut salad greens. Yes, it's expensive, but it's good and easy.

- If you just won't take any time to cut up vegetables for salads and are willing to pay a premium for someone else to do the work, then take advantage of the supermarket salad bar. Buy enough at the salad bar to add up to a few salads for the week.

12 EXCELLENT SOURCES OF VITAMIN A

Food	Serving Size	% Daily Value
Carrot juice	1/2 cup	633%
Pumpkin, cooked*	1/2 cup	542%
Carrots, whole	1 medium	405%
Sweet potatoes, yams, cooked*	1/2 cup	389%
Squash*: butternut, hubbard, winter, acorn, cooked	1/2 cup	288%
Spinach, kale, cooked	1/2 cup	122%
Greens: beet, collard, mustard, turnip, cooked	1/2 cup	35–73%
Bok choy, cooked	1/2 cup	48%
Watercress, raw	1 cup	32%
Red pepper, raw	1/2 cup	28%
Tomato paste	3 Tbsp	24%
Broccoli, cooked	1/2 cup	23%

*Vegetables found in the starch group.

- Top salads with these less-than-usual vegetables: beets, carrots, raw broccoli, and red, green, or yellow peppers. They're terrific sources of nutrition and add variety to salads.

Dress with Less

The calories from regular salad dressing add up quickly. Just two tablespoons of Thousand Island or blue cheese dressing can add 150 calories of fat. Even the calories from reduced-fat, low-fat, and fat-free dressing add up quickly. The challenge with salads is to pick your salad dressing carefully and tip the bottle gingerly.

11 EXCELLENT SOURCES OF VITAMIN C

Food	Serving Size	% Daily Value
Red pepper, raw	1/2 cup	158%
Broccoli, cooked	1/2 cup	97%
Hot chili peppers, raw	2 Tbsp	75%
Green peppers, raw	1/2 cup	75%
Kohlrabi, cooked	1/2 cup	75%
Kale, cooked	1/2 cup	67%
Cabbage, green and red, raw	1 cup	48–67%
Snow peas, cooked	1/2 cup	63%
Bok choy, raw	1 cup	53%
Cauliflower, cooked	1/2 cup	47%
Tomatoes, tomato juice	1 serving	33%

FOLATE: ESSENTIAL TO GOOD HEALTH

Folate, one of the B vitamins, has been linked to the prevention of heart attacks, stroke, and colon and rectal cancer, and birth defects such as spina bifida.

Folate is found in many fruits and vegetables. Other foods such as enriched grain products, breakfast cereals, infant formulas, and medical foods, foods for special dietary use, and meal-replacement products are fortified with folate.

Adult men and women need 400 micrograms of folate (also known as folic acid or folacin) in their diet each day. By eating at least 5 servings of fruits and vegetables a day, dried peas and beans several times a week, and fortified grain products, you'll get enough folate.

10 EXCELLENT SOURCES OF FOLATE

Food	Serving Size	% Daily Value
Spinach, cooked	1/2 cup	34%
Okra, cooked	1 cup	34%
Beets, cooked, from raw	1/2 cup	30%
Turnip greens, cooked	1/2 cup	21%
Romaine lettuce	1 cup	19%
Chinese cabbage and bok choy, raw	1 cup	11-18%
Bean sprouts, raw	1 cup	16%
Artichoke	1 globe	15%
Mustard greens, cooked	1/2 cup	12%
Broccoli, cooked	1/2 cup	11%

Other excellent vegetable sources of folate are dried peas and beans (from the starch group) and soy-based products (in the meat and meat substitutes group).

Here are the nutrition numbers on Thousand Island and Italian dressing in regular, low-fat, and fat-free:

Serving: 2 Tbsp	Calories	Carbohydrate (g)	Fat (g)
Regular			
Thousand Island	118	5	11
Italian	183	2	20
Low-calorie			
Thousand Island	48	5	3
Italian	32	2	3
Fat-free			
Thousand Island	20	6	0
Italian	18	4	0

Tips to Dress with Less

Try several salad dressings and find a few you enjoy. You might settle on a regular dressing and then use just a small amount or dilute it with vinegar. Or you might find that a homemade dressing with olive, canola, or walnut oil (which are all high in "good" monounsaturated fats) suits you best. When you eat away from home and you can't get a lower-fat dressing, try these tips:

- Order salad dressing on the side. This puts you in control of the amount that is ladled on your salad.
- Try the fork-and-dip technique. Some people find they use less if they just dip forkfuls of salad in the dressing.
- Ask for vinegar or lemon wedges on the side to dilute a small amount of dressing and spread it over the salad.

3 Flavored Vinegars

Serving Size: 1 Tbsp, Total Servings: 32

To cut down even further on excess fat intake, why not enjoy a salad with just a good splash of aromatic, flavored vinegar? It's fun to make your own flavored vinegars, and you can even give these as gifts. Also splash into soups, sauces, and stews to wake up the flavor. All recipes make 1 pint, with 10 minutes preparation time.

For all of the vinegars, put the ingredients into tall decorative bottles. Let stand in a cool, dark place for about 1 month.

Herb Vinegar

- 1 pint white wine vinegar
- 1 sprig fresh thyme
- 1 sprig fresh rosemary
- 1 sprig fresh marjoram
- 2 cloves garlic
- 1 sprig fresh thyme

Berry Vinegar

- 1 pint white wine vinegar
- 1/2 cup fresh raspberries or blackberries
- 2 Tbsp honey
- 1 cinnamon stick

Spicy Vinegar

- 1 pint white wine vinegar
- 1 Tbsp black peppercorns
- 2 chili peppers
- 1 garlic clove
- 1/4 tsp ground ginger

Exchanges, Herb Vinegar & Spicy Vinegar
Free food

Calories	1
Calories from Fat	0
Total Fat	0 g
Saturated Fat	0 g
Cholesterol	0 mg
Sodium	0 mg
Carbohydrate	1 g
Dietary Fiber	0 g
Sugars	0 g
Protein	0 g

Exchanges, Berry Vinegar
Free food

Calories	5
Calories from Fat	0
Total Fat	0 g
Saturated Fat	0 g
Cholesterol	0 mg
Sodium	0 mg
Carbohydrate	2 g
Dietary Fiber	0 g
Sugars	1 g
Protein	0 g

5 Easy Dressings (with Low-fat Sour Cream)

Serving Size: 2 Tbsp, Total Servings: 12

We use a low-fat sour cream instead of a fat-free one. We tested several fat-free ones and found that the low-fat had a more pleasing taste. Sour cream dressings are rich and thick and will really remind you of a decadent high-fat dressing.

Basic Dressing

1 cup low-fat sour cream	**2–3** Tbsp fat-free milk or butter-milk
1/2 cup low-fat mayonnaise	**2** tsp red wine vinegar
1/2 tsp fresh ground pepper	

1 Combine all ingredients by hand until smooth, and add one of the Variation Ingredients. Preparation time: 5 minutes.

Variations:

Herb:
Add 1 tsp minced herbs (any)

Salsa:
Add 1/4 cup of salsa

Cheese:
Add 3 Tbsp crumbled blue cheese

Curry:
Add 1 tsp curry powder

Orange:
Add 2 Tbsp orange juice, omit vinegar

Exchanges, Herb Variation
1/2 Starch

Calories	41
Calories from Fat	21
Total Fat	2 g
Saturated Fat	1 g
Cholesterol	7 mg
Sodium	108 mg
Carbohydrate	4 g
Dietary Fiber	0 g
Sugars	3 g
Protein	1 g

Exchanges, Cheese Variation
1/2 Starch

Calories	49
Calories from Fat	27
Total Fat	3 g
Saturated Fat	1 g
Cholesterol	8 mg
Sodium	140 mg
Carbohydrate	4 g
Dietary Fiber	0 g
Sugars	3 g
Protein	2 g

Allium Vegetables

Members of the allium family, which include garlic, chives, onions, leeks, and shallots, contain the phytochemical allicin. It has been suggested, though not proven, that allicin might help lower cholesterol, decrease the incidence of cancers of the gastrointestinal tract, and help control blood pressure. Onions are also a good source of vitamin C.

Many of the recipes in this book use garlic and onions. Adding their flavor helps you cut down on fat. Roasted garlic, for example, is a great substitute for fat on potatoes, bread, and pasta.

Tomatoes: Vitamin C and More

Tomatoes and tomato products are a good source of vitamin A and an excellent source of vitamin C. One ripe tomato picked from the garden gives you about 20 milligrams of vitamin C—one-third the Reference Daily Intake for vitamin C.

Tomatoes and tomato products also offer lycopene, the pigment that gives the ripe tomato its bright red color. It's one of a family of natural pigments called carotenoids.

Some studies suggest that lycopene may slow the development of cancer of the prostate, digestive tract, breast, lung, and cervix, as well as protect against heart disease.

Some studies show particular benefit from the lycopene in tomato products, such as stewed tomatoes, and tomato sauce, paste, and ketchup, rather than raw tomatoes, because the lycopene is absorbed more efficiently.

How to Buy: For fresh tomatoes, purchase plump, unblemished tomatoes. Never buy tomatoes that have been refrigerated, because that ruins the flavor. Try to wait for vine-ripened tomatoes in the summer and fall.

Keep a can of tomatoes on hand. (Look for no-salt-added.) They add flavor to cooked rice, pasta, and many other dishes. With canned tomatoes, you have your choice of whole, diced, puréed, or crushed. Look for cans without dents or rust.

How to Store: Keep tomatoes at room temperature and use within 2–3 days.

Uses: Add tomatoes to salads, soups, stews, and main dishes. Use canned tomatoes when fresh are not at their peak.

Roasted Garlic

Serving Size: 2 cloves, Total Servings: 10

Get the heart-healthy benefits of garlic in a more subtle way than just eating raw garlic. Roasting garlic will mellow its strong taste so you can eat more of it. You don't even need special garlic bakers to make this.

1 large head garlic

1 sprig fresh rosemary

1/4 cup fat-free, reduced-sodium chicken broth

1 tsp olive oil

1 Preheat the oven to 375°F. Cut a medium square of aluminum foil.

2 Cut a slice off the top of the garlic just to expose the top of the cloves. Put the garlic in the center of the foil. Top with the rosemary sprig. Pour the broth and olive oil over the garlic.

3 Bring all four corners of the foil together and twist to seal. Place on a small baking sheet. Bake for 1 hour until the garlic is soft.

4 To eat: Open the foil. Put the garlic on a small dish. Peel a clove away from the bulb. Squeeze the garlic from its skin and spread on bread, potatoes, pasta, vegetables, and more!

PREPARATION
5 minutes

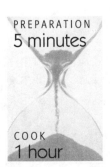

COOK
1 hour

Exchanges
Free food

Calories 12
  Calories from Fat 4
Total Fat . . . . 0 g
  Saturated Fat . . . . 0 g
Cholesterol . . . . 0 mg
Sodium . . . . 14 mg
Carbohydrate . . . . 2 g
  Dietary Fiber . . . . 0 g
  Sugars . . . . 2 g
Protein . . . . 0 g

Caramelized Onions

Serving Size: 2 Tbsp, Total Servings: 40

Use these delicious onions to toss into pasta, add to an omelette, top a baked potato or homemade pizza, or add to cooked vegetables instead of butter and heavy, fat-laden sauces.

1/2 cup water

8 cups thinly sliced yellow onions

2 Tbsp sugar

1 In a large skillet over medium high heat, heat the water to a simmer. Add the onions, cover, and let cook for 45 minutes. As water evaporates, keep adding more throughout the 45 minutes.

2 Uncover and lower the heat to simmer. Add the sugar and continue to cook, adding more water if necessary for about another 45 minutes until onions are richly brown.

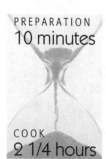

PREPARATION
10 minutes

COOK
2 1/4 hours

Exchanges
Free food

Calories	15
Calories from Fat	1
Total Fat	0 g
Saturated Fat	0 g
Cholesterol	0 mg
Sodium	1 mg
Carbohydrate	3 g
Dietary Fiber	1 g
Sugars	3 g
Protein	0 g

Green Beans with Tomatoes and Herbs

Serving Size: about 3/4 cup, Total Servings: 4

The sauce for this recipe can be used as an all-around basic tomato sauce. Substitute zucchini, asparagus, or broccoli for the green beans if you like.

1 Tbsp olive oil	1 tsp minced basil
2 cloves garlic, minced	1 tsp minced oregano
1 small onion, minced	1 lb trimmed green beans
1 can (14-oz) crushed tomatoes	Salt and pepper to taste

1 In a medium skillet over medium heat, heat the oil. Add the garlic and onion and sauté for 5 minutes. Add the tomatoes, basil, and oregano. Cook for 2 minutes.

2 Add the green beans. Cover and cook for 6 minutes. Season with salt and pepper.

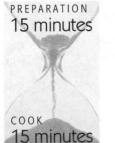

PREPARATION
15 minutes

COOK
15 minutes

Exchanges
3 Vegetable   1 Fat
(3 Vegetable = 1 Carbohydrate)

Calories 113
    Calories from Fat 32
Total Fat . . . . .4 g
    Saturated Fat . . . . .1 g
Cholesterol . . . . .0 mg
Sodium . . . . .281 mg
Carbohydrate . . . . .18 g
    Dietary Fiber . . . . .6 g
    Sugars . . . . .8 g
Protein . . . . .4 g

Zucchini Marinara

Serving Size: about 1/2 cup, Total Servings: 4

Starting with fresh tomatoes will make your sauce much more flavorful than canned tomatoes. If you can find tomatoes still on the vine, the better flavored they will be. Use asparagus, broccoli, spinach, or cabbage as a substitute for the zucchini if desired.

2	tsp olive oil	**1**	Tbsp minced basil
1	small onion, thinly sliced	**1 1/2**	cups sliced zucchini
2	medium tomatoes, chopped		Salt and pepper to taste
2	cloves garlic, minced	**1**	Tbsp Parmesan cheese
1	Tbsp minced fresh parsley		

1 In a skillet over medium heat, heat the oil. Add the onion and sauté for 4 minutes.

2 Add the tomatoes, garlic, parsley, and basil. Cook for 3 minutes.

3 Add the zucchini and cook for 5 minutes. Season with salt and pepper and sprinkle with Parmesan.

PREPARATION
10 minutes

COOK
about 12 minutes

Exchanges
2 Vegetable
1/2 Fat

Calories	60
Calories from Fat	27
Total Fat	3 g
Saturated Fat	1 g
Cholesterol	2 mg
Sodium	42 mg
Carbohydrate	8 g
Dietary Fiber	2 g
Sugars	5 g
Protein	2 g

Cruciferous Vegetables

Cruciferous vegetables are named for their cross- (crucifer) shaped flowers. The group includes broccoli, Brussels sprouts, cabbage, cauliflower, collards, kale, kohlrabi, rutabagas, turnips, and turnip greens. Cruciferous vegetables may guard against some cancers, so eat one of the many cruciferous vegetables two to three times a week.

Certain cruciferous vegetables really shine. Broccoli is an excellent source of vitamins A and C and a good source of folate.

How to Buy and Store

Broccoli: Sold year-round. Choose crisp, uniformly green heads with tight clusters that have not begun to flower or yellow. The stems should not be too thick. Store in plastic bags and use within a few days.

Brussels sprouts: Sold loose or in packages. Choose firm, compact, bright-green sprouts with no signs of yellowing. Put in a plastic bag and use within a few days.

Cabbage: Choose cabbage heads that are firm, heavy for their size, and free of yellowing leaves. Tight cabbage heads will stay in the refrigerator for two weeks.

Cauliflower: Choose clean, compact heads with fresh-looking, light-green leaves and creamy white florets. Tightly wrap in plastic and use within one week.

Uses

Broccoli, cabbage, and cauliflower can be eaten raw as well as cooked. Brussels sprouts are eaten cooked. Use as vegetable side dishes; as part of casseroles, one-pot meals, and soups; on raw vegetable plates; and to top pasta, rice, or potatoes.

Dark, Leafy Greens

With dark, leafy greens, you get vitamins A and C, and several in the group also offer some calcium and folate. For example, spinach is an excellent source of vitamin A and folate, and a good source of vitamin C and iron. Kale is an excellent source of vitamins A and C.

How to Buy: Look for fresh-looking leaves and stems. Avoid leaves that are wilted or yellowing, or have insect holes.

How to Store: Store in plastic bags with breather holes. Most dark, leafy greens should be used within 1 to 3 days. Wash the greens well before use as many of them are quite sandy and gritty.

Uses: Dark, leafy greens can be eaten raw or cooked. Whenever you can, eat them raw or lightly cooked to preserve all the nutrients.

Broccoli with Sesame Seeds and Scallions

Serving Size: about 1/2 cup, Total Servings: 4

Broccoli should be cooked just until the color becomes bright green. There is nothing more distasteful than army-green color and limp broccoli! Our favorite method is blanching (see below). You can also steam your broccoli on the stovetop or microwave it, just make sure it comes out crunchy and beautiful.

1 1/2 lbs broccoli (generally about 1 large bundle). Peel the stems if necessary and slice into 1/2-inch slices. Cut the broccoli into florets.

6 cups water

2 cloves garlic, minced

3 scallions, minced

2 Tbsp rice vinegar

2 tsp sesame oil

1 Tbsp sesame seeds

1 In a large pot, boil the water and then add the broccoli. Boil 1 minute and turn off the heat.

2 Drain the broccoli, put broccoli into a bowl of cold water, and then drain again.

3 In a large bowl, combine the garlic, scallions, vinegar, sesame oil, and sesame seeds. Add the broccoli and toss well. Serve at room temperature.

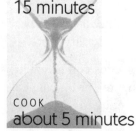

PREPARATION
15 minutes

COOK
about 5 minutes

Exchanges
2 Vegetable
1/2 Fat

Calories 69
   Calories from Fat 34
Total Fat . . . . 4 g
   Saturated Fat . . . . 1 g
Cholesterol . . . . 0 mg
Sodium . . . . 31 mg
Carbohydrate . . . . 8 g
   Dietary Fiber . . . . 4 g
   Sugars . . . . 3 g
Protein . . . . 4 g

Broccoli and Garlic

Serving Size: 1/2 cup, Total Servings: 4

This time, garlic is sliced into thin slivers. By not mincing the garlic finely, the garlic flavor of this dish is heightened. In every bite a pungent slice of garlic will delight your taste buds.

2 tsp peanut oil	**1/2** cup fat-free, reduced-sodium chicken broth
3 cloves garlic, sliced	**2** tsp toasted sesame seeds
1 tsp minced ginger	Salt and pepper
2 cups broccoli florets	

1 In a wok, heat the oil over medium heat. Add the garlic and ginger and sauté for 30 seconds.

2 Add the broccoli and broth, cover, and steam for 3–4 minutes. Top with sesame seeds and season with salt and pepper.

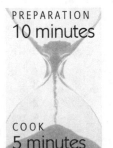

PREPARATION
10 minutes

COOK
5 minutes

Exchanges
1 Vegetable
1/2 Fat

Calories 42
   Calories from Fat 28
Total Fat . . . . 3 g
   Saturated Fat . . . . 1 g
Cholesterol . . . . 0 mg
Sodium . . . . 25 mg
Carbohydrate . . . . 3 g
   Dietary Fiber . . . . 1 g
   Sugars . . . . 2 g
Protein . . . . 2 g

Brussels Sprouts with Chestnuts

Serving Size: 1/2 cup, Total Servings: 4

This is our favorite way to prepare Brussels sprouts, especially around holiday time. The earthy chestnuts provide a nice contrast to the slightly peppery flavor of the Brussels sprouts. Chestnuts are available canned, which is easier than having to roast and peel them.

2	cups Brussels sprouts	**1**	green onion, minced
2	tsp olive oil		Salt and pepper
1/2	cup cooked canned chestnuts		Nutmeg
1/3	cup chicken broth		

1 Prepare the Brussels sprouts. Wash them and then cut an X in the bottom of each sprout.

2 In a large saucepan, bring 1 inch of water to a boil. Add the sprouts, return to a boil, cover, and cook for 6–7 minutes. Drain.

3 In a large skillet over medium heat, heat the oil. Add the chestnuts and sauté for 1 minute. Add the sprouts and cook for 1 minute. Add the broth and cover and cook for 1 minute. Add the scallion, salt, pepper, and nutmeg and cook for 1 minute.

PREPARATION
10 minutes

COOK
10 minutes

Exchanges
1/2 Starch
2 Vegetable

Calories	99
Calories from Fat	24
Total Fat	3 g
Saturated Fat	0 g
Cholesterol	0 mg
Sodium	57 mg
Carbohydrate	18 g
Dietary Fiber	2 g
Sugars	5 g
Protein	3 g

Cauliflower with Cheddar Cheese Sauce

Serving Size: 3/4 cup cauliflower, about 1/2 cup sauce,
Total Servings: 4

Cauliflower with cheese sauce has been a favorite for many for so long. Fortunately, with reduced-fat milk and lower-fat cheese, you can still have the creamy, rich taste of a sauce blanketing perfectly cooked, snow-white cauliflower. Be sure the cheese is finely grated, and add it to the sauce in small amounts. Adding large chunks will make the sauce glob. This sauce can also be used to top any vegetable or a baked potato, blanket cooked chicken or fish, or add to pasta or rice.

1 whole medium head cauliflower, outer green leaves removed, stem trimmed

Sauce

1/4 cup all-purpose flour

2 cups 1% milk

1 cup finely grated low-fat cheddar cheese

1 Tbsp grated Parmesan cheese

Fresh ground black pepper

1 Steam the cauliflower: Set a steamer basket in 2 inches of water in a pot large enough to hold the whole head. Set the head on the basket and cover. (If head protrudes, use a piece of foil instead of the lid.) Bring the water to a rolling boil and boil for 15-20 minutes until cauliflower is cooked through yet tender. Remove the cauliflower from the pot and drain.

2 To prepare the cheese sauce: In a medium skillet over medium heat, add the flour. Stir the flour for 1 minute. Slowly add the milk to the flour, whisking constantly. Keep whisking until sauce thickens. This should take about 10 minutes.

3 Remove the sauce from the heat. Slowly add the cheese, whisking after each addition. Grind in pepper. Serve the cheese sauce poured over the cauliflower and then serve by separating into florets.

PREPARATION
10 minutes

COOK
30 minutes

Exchanges
1 1/2 Carbohydrate
1 Lean Meat

Calories 171
   Calories from Fat 38
Total Fat . . . . 4 g
   Saturated Fat . . . . 2 g
Cholesterol . . . . 13 mg
Sodium . . . . 310 mg
Carbohydrate . . . . 20 g
   Dietary Fiber . . . . 4 g
   Sugars . . . . 9 g
Protein . . . . 15 g

Curried Cauliflower Soup

Serving Size: about 1 1/4 cups, Total Servings: 4

This soup has a brilliant color from the curry. Always use a russet potato when making soups. The russet potato has the ideal starch content to hold its shape during soup making.

2 tsp canola oil

1 small onion, diced

2 cloves garlic, minced

3/4 tsp curry powder

3/4 lb cauliflower florets, coarsely chopped

1 medium russet potato, peeled and diced

2 cups 1% milk

2 cups fat-free, reduced-sodium chicken broth

Salt and pepper to taste

1 In a stockpot over medium heat, heat the oil. Add the onion and garlic and sauté for 2 minutes. Add the curry powder and sauté for 30 seconds.

2 Add the cauliflower and potato to the pan. Add the milk and broth and lower the heat to simmer. Cook, partially covered on low for 20 minutes.

3 Transfer the contents of the stockpot to a blender (in two batches if necessary). Puree the soup until smooth. Season with salt and pepper.

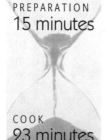

PREPARATION
15 minutes

COOK
23 minutes

Exchanges
1 1/2 Carbohydrate
1/2 Fat

Calories 140
  Calories from Fat 35
Total Fat . . . . .4 g
  Saturated Fat . . . . .1 g
Cholesterol . . . . .5 mg
Sodium . . . . .330 mg
Carbohydrate . . . . .19 g
  Dietary Fiber . . . . .3 g
  Sugars . . . . .10 g
Protein . . . . .8 g

Healthy Coleslaw
Serving Size: 1/2 cup, Total Servings: 8

Most people don't realize that cabbage is a very nutritious food. Making coleslaw is probably the easiest way to get its cancer-fighting properties.

Dressing

- **1** cup non-fat plain yogurt
- **1/4** cup apple cider vinegar
- **1** Tbsp honey

Slaw

- **1** lb (1 small head) green cabbage, shredded
- **1/2** cup shredded carrot
- **1** Tbsp poppy seeds
- **1/4** cup raisins or currants

1 In a large bowl, combine the dressing ingredients. Add the cabbage, carrots, poppy seeds, and raisins. Mix well until the dressing completely coats the cabbage.

PREPARATION
20 minutes

Exchanges
1 Carbohydrate

Calories 58
Calories from Fat 6
Total Fat . . . . 1 g
Saturated Fat . . . . 0 g
Cholesterol . . . . 1 mg
Sodium . . . . 36 mg
Carbohydrate . . . . 12 g
Dietary Fiber . . . . 2 g
Sugars . . . . 9 g
Protein . . . . 3 g

Fall Spinach Salad

Serving Size: about 3/4 cup, Total Servings: 4

Even on a low-fat food plan, you can still enjoy the tastes of high-fat foods when you use them in small quantities. The sharp flavor of blue cheese combines well with lower-fat mayonnaise, and you get the best of both worlds. Granny Smith apples have a nice tart, yet somewhat sweet taste that goes well with the cheese in the dressing.

Salad

- **1** lb fresh spinach leaves, washed, stemmed, and torn
- **1** small red onion, sliced very thinly into rings
- **1** large Granny Smith apple, unpeeled and chopped into 1/4-inch cubes
- **2** Tbsp toasted walnuts

Dressing

- **1/2** cup fat-free sour cream
- **1/2** cup low-fat mayonnaise
- **1/4** cup red wine vinegar
- **2** cloves garlic, minced
- **1/3** cup crumbled blue cheese

1 Combine all the salad ingredients in a large salad bowl.

2 In a small bowl, whisk the sour cream, mayonnaise, red wine vinegar, and garlic. Add the blue cheese.

3 Serve salad dressing with the spinach salad.

PREPARATION
20 minutes

Exchanges
2 Carbohydrate
1 1/2 Fat

Calories 208
Calories from Fat 73
Total Fat . . . . 8 g
Saturated Fat . . . . 2 g
Cholesterol . . . . 10 mg
Sodium . . . . 556 mg
Carbohydrate . . . . 29 g
Dietary Fiber . . . . 5 g
Sugars . . . . 17 g
Protein . . . . 7 g

Soy Kale

Serving Size: about 1 cup, Total Servings: 4

Kale deserves better treatment than just using it as a garnish on a dinner plate. You don't need gobs of fat to enhance its flavor. Asian ingredients of ginger and soy bring out the best in kale.

2 lbs fresh kale	**3** cloves garlic, minced
2 tsp sesame oil	**2** Tbsp lite soy sauce
2 tsp minced ginger	

1 To prepare the kale, first wash the leaves in several changes of water until the water runs clear. Remove the leaf part from the tough stem and discard the stem. Tear the kale coarsely. Do not pat dry.

2 In a large heavy skillet or wok, heat the oil over medium high heat. Add the ginger and garlic and sauté for 1 minute. Add the kale with the water still clinging to the leaves from washing.

3 Sauté for 1 minute and then cover and steam for 2 minutes until kale is softened. Add the soy sauce and serve.

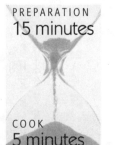

PREPARATION
15 minutes

COOK
5 minutes

Exchanges
2 Vegetable
1/2 Fat

Calories 77
Calories from Fat 27
Total Fat . . . . 3 g
Saturated Fat . . . . 0 g
Cholesterol . . . . 0 mg
Sodium . . . . 340 mg
Carbohydrate . . . . .10 g
Dietary Fiber . . . . 3 g
Sugars . . . . 5 g
Protein . . . . 3 g

Arugula and Watercress Salad

Serving Size: 1 cup, Total Servings: 4

This is an assertive salad. The slightly peppery taste of the arugula and watercress is balanced with the sweet oranges and an orange dressing. We would serve this for dinner parties as well as for everyday dining.

2 cups torn, washed arugula leaves

2 cups washed watercress leaves, stemmed

1 orange, peeled, sectioned, seeded, and chopped

2 Tbsp toasted almond slivers

Dressing

2 Tbsp olive oil

1/4 cup orange juice

1/2 tsp grated orange zest

2 tsp lemon juice

Salt and pepper to taste

1 Combine the arugula, watercress, orange, and almonds in a large salad bowl.

2 Whisk together the olive oil, orange juice, zest, and lemon juice in a small bowl. Add salt and pepper to taste. Pour over the salad and serve.

PREPARATION
20 minutes

Exchanges
1/2 Fruit
1 1/2 Fat

Calories 108
   Calories from Fat 74
Total Fat . . . . 8 g
   Saturated Fat . . . . 1 g
Cholesterol . . . . 0 mg
Sodium . . . . 11 mg
Carbohydrate . . . . 8 g
   Dietary Fiber . . . . 2 g
   Sugars . . . . 5 g
Protein . . . . 2 g

Spinach Sauté with Mushrooms

Serving Size: about 1/2 cup, Total Servings: 4

Fresh spinach is always a little dirty, so be sure to rinse it well. Steam the spinach until it is just wilted, but still nice and bright green.

2 Tbsp olive oil	3 bunches spinach (about 2 lbs), stemmed and washed
2 cloves garlic, minced	
1 cup mushrooms, sliced	1 Tbsp lemon juice
	Salt and pepper to taste

1 In a skillet over medium heat, heat the oil. Add the mushrooms and garlic and sauté for 3 minutes.

2 Add the spinach, cover, and steam for 2 minutes. Add the lemon juice, salt, and pepper. Serve immediately.

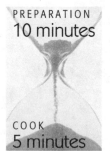

PREPARATION
10 minutes

COOK
5 minutes

Exchanges
1 Vegetable
1 1/2 Fat

Calories 99
   Calories from Fat 60
Total Fat . . . . 7 g
   Saturated Fat . . . . 1 g
Cholesterol . . . . 0 mg
Sodium . . . . 132 mg
Carbohydrate . . . . 7 g
   Dietary Fiber . . . . 5 g
   Sugars . . . . 1 g
Protein . . . . 5 g

	Exchange/ Serving	Calories	Carbohydrate (g)	Protein (g)	Fiber (g)
Artichoke, cooked	1/2	30	7	2	3
Artichoke hearts	1/2 cup	36	7	2	0
Asparagus, frozen	1/2 cup	23	4	2	3
Asparagus spears, canned, drained	1/2 cup	23	3	3	2
Beans (green, wax), canned, drained	1/2 cup	14	3	1	1
Beans, snap, frozen	1/2 cup	18	4	1	2
Bean sprouts, raw	1 cup	31	6	3	2
Beets, canned, sliced, drained	1/2 cup	26	6	1	2
Broccoli, raw, chopped	1 cup	25	5	3	3
Broccoli spears, frozen	1/2 cup	26	5	3	3
Brussels sprouts, frozen, cooked	1/2 cup	33	6	3	3
Cabbage, cooked	1/2 cup	16	3	1	2
Cabbage, Chinese, raw	1 cup	12	2	1	1
Cabbage, green, raw	1 cup	18	4	1	2
Carrots, canned, drained	1/2 cup	17	4	0	1
Carrots, cooked	1/2 cup	35	8	1	3
Carrots, raw	1 cup	47	11	1	3
Cauliflower, frozen, cooked	1/2 cup	17	3	1	2
Cauliflower, raw	1 cup	25	5	2	2
Celery, cooked	1/2 cup	14	3	1	1
Celery, raw	1 cup	19	4	1	2
Cucumber, raw	1 cup	14	3	1	1
Eggplant, cooked	1/2 cup	13	3	0	1
Endive/escarole, raw	1 cup	9	2	1	2
Greens, cooked					
Collard	1/2 cup	17	4	1	1
Kale	1/2 cup	21	4	1	1
Mustard	1/2 cup	10	2	2	1
Turnip	1/2 cup	14	3	1	2
Kohlrabi, cooked	1/2 cup	24	6	2	1
Lettuce, iceberg	1 cup	7	1	1	1

Vegetables

	Exchange/ Serving	Calories	Carbohydrate (g)	Protein (g)	Fiber (g)
Mixed vegetables (no corn, peas, pasta)	1/2 cup	20	3	1	1
Mushrooms, canned, drained	1/2 cup	19	4	2	2
Mushrooms, fresh, cooked	1/2 cup	21	4	2	2
Mushrooms, raw	1 cup	18	3	2	1
Okra, frozen, cooked	1/2 cup	34	8	2	3
Onions, chopped, cooked	1/2 cup	46	11	1	2
Onions, raw	1 cup	61	14	2	3
Onion, green, raw	1 cup	32	7	2	3
Pea pods, cooked	1/2 cup	34	6	3	2
Pea pods, raw	1 cup	61	11	4	4
Pepper, green, cooked	1/2 cup	19	5	1	1
Pepper, green, raw	1 cup	27	6	1	2
Pepper, hot green chile, raw	1 cup	60	14	3	2
Radishes	1 cup	20	4	1	2
Romaine	1 cup	9	1	1	1
Sauerkraut, canned (sodium)	1/2 cup	22	5	1	3
Spinach, canned, drained	1/2 cup	25	4	3	3
Spinach, frozen, cooked	1/2 cup	27	5	3	3
Spinach, raw	1 cup	12	2	2	2
Squash, summer, cooked	1/2 cup	18	4	1	1
Squash, summer, raw	1 cup	26	6	2	2
Tomatoes, canned, solids and liquids	1/2 cup	24	5	1	1
Tomatoes, raw	1 cup	38	8	2	2
Tomato juice (sodium)	1/2 cup	21	5	1	0
Tomato sauce (sodium)	1/2 cup	37	9	2	2
Turnips, cooked, cubed	1/2 cup	14	4	1	2
Vegetable juice (sodium)	1/2 cup	23	6	1	1
Water chestnuts	1/2 cup	35	9	1	2
Watercress, raw	1 cup	4	0	1	0
Zucchini, raw	1 cup	18	4	2	2
Zucchini squash, sliced, cooked	1/2 cup	14	4	1	1

(sodium) = 400 mg or more of sodium per exchange.

FOCUS ON Water

Do you feel tired? Do you get headaches?
The cure may be easier than you would
ever guess: Drink more water.

Water is often overlooked as a nutrient, but it is essential. A shortage of water will affect your health more quickly than a shortage of any other nutrient.

You need roughly 8 to 12 cups of fluids a day to keep well hydrated. Some of your fluid needs are met through food, particularly fruits and vegetables, as they contain a high percentage of water. The rest you need to drink. Eight 8-ounce glasses a day should give you enough fluids.

Just plain water is often overlooked, but it is the best bet to meet your need for fluids. It's available, inexpensive, and has no calories. What could be better? Opt for water whenever you have the choice. Keep water nearby so that you think to drink before you get thirsty.

■ Keep a plastic container filled with water by your desk. Sip water throughout the day.

■ Fill a water bottle and take it with you on errands, weekend family outings, and sporting events.

■ Buy bottled water instead of automatically choosing soda or juice. Luckily over the last few years bottled water has become more commonplace. It's no longer unusual to see water sold at a baseball game or a food court.

■ Drink water at meals. Even if you drink another beverage, keep a glass of water by your side so you drink more water.

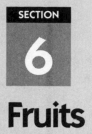

SECTION

6

Fruits

RECIPES

Blueberries with Almond Cream _____ 131

Blueberry Lemon Muffins _____ 132

Strawberry-Peach Soup _____ 133

Strawberry Raspberry Almond Shake _____ 134

Orange and Fennel Salad _____ 135

Grapefruit Combo Salad _____ 136

Lime Guacamole with Mango _____ 138

Pan-Seared Pork with Mango Salsa _____ 139

Mango Chicken Salad _____ 140

Cool Melon Soup _____ 141

Orange and Kiwi Salad _____ 142

Minted Kiwi Salad _____ 143

Apple Sandwiches _____ 146

Red Cherry Frozen Yogurt Sundae _____ 147

Red Grape and Turkey Salad _____ 148

Pears Baked with White Wine _____ 149

Island Sundaes _____ 150

6 Fruits

Fruits are packed with vitamins and minerals, they satisfy your sweet tooth, and many make great portable snacks or put the finishing touch to a meal.

A serving or exchange of fruit contains about 15 grams of carbohydrate, nearly all as sucrose, and about 60 calories. In general, a fruit exchange or serving is 1 small-to-medium fresh fruit, 1/2 cup canned fruit or fruit juice, or 1/4 cup dried fruit.

The diabetes food pyramid suggests you eat 2 to 4 servings of fruits each day. Just as with vegetables, you'll want to eat a variety so you get a wide spectrum of vitamins, minerals, phytochemicals, and antioxidants.

Look at your current habits. If at best you average 1 or 2 servings of fruits per day, first work towards increasing that to 2 or 3. Then down the road, ratchet the number up 1 more if need be.

Here's how easily you can fit in 3 servings of fruit a day: For breakfast, have a small banana on your cereal; for a midday snack have a kiwi; and for dessert that evening, 1 1/4 cups whole strawberries sliced on frozen yogurt. The next day, have 1/2 cup orange juice at breakfast (make sure it's 100% unsweetened juice), an apple with your lunch, and 1/2 cup mango with plain yogurt after dinner.

Fit in Fruit

Here are easy ways to add fruit (and its bounty of vitamins and minerals)
to your meals:

- Keep your refrigerator stocked with fresh fruit. If it's there, you're more likely to eat it.
- Take one or two pieces of fruit with you to work. It's so hard to find fruit when you eat out and if you do it's so pricey you won't buy it. This way you have it with you, and it's easy to eat a piece after lunch or as a snack.
- Think about eating a piece of fruit on the way home to keep you from walking in the door and eating everything that isn't nailed down.
- Keep fruit at the ready. Cut up a bunch of fruit—oranges, kiwi, cantaloupe, mango, grapefruit, grapes—and keep in a plastic container. Eat a serving plain or topped with nonfat yogurt (plain or fruited) at breakfast or as an afternoon or evening snack.
- If you don't have the time or desire to cut up fruit, buy cut-up fruit in the super-market. In some supermarkets it's at the deli counter and in others it's at the salad bar.
- Keep canned fruit and dried fruit in your cupboard, and frozen unsweetened fruit in your freezer. They are good for a long time and come in handy when you run out of fresh fruit.
- Work a serving of fruit into breakfast: fruit on cold cereal; hot cereal cooked with raisins, apricots, or cut-up prunes; a portable banana as you walk out the door.
- Think of fruit toppings for salads: raisins, dried cranberries, pineapple chunks, pieces of mango, kiwi, or apples.
- Toss fruit into casseroles, meat loaf, or sauces: dried apricots in a rice casserole, raisins in meat loaf, or blueberries in maple syrup.
- Blend maple or table syrup with no-sugar-added applesauce.
- Put blueberries, raspberries, strawberries, or other fruits in the blender to make a topping for frozen yogurt, ice cream, plain yogurt, or cake.
- Pack raisins or other dried fruit into lunch boxes, keep them in a desk drawer for snacks, and take them on day-long activities, such as skiing or hiking.

EAT MORE, BUT...

The message above is certainly Eat More Fruit. However, there's an important
"But" that goes along with that message: *But* be aware of how much you're eating.

It's easy to eat more fruit than you realize. One fruit exchange equals one *small*
apple, one *small* orange, or one *medium* peach, each of which has about 60
calories. Those aren't the sizes you find in the supermarket. An average apple or
pear in the supermarket today is at least 80 calories and often tops 100 calories. If

your meal plan calls for 1 fruit exchange and you eat a large apple, your blood glucose may go higher than you expected. If you regularly eat more fruit than you realize, you may gain weight.

Tips for Portion Control

- At the grocery store, remind yourself that biggest is not necessarily the best. Choose small pieces of fruit.
- Review the serving sizes of fresh fruits on page 151. Then use the scales in the produce area of your supermarket. Find out what a 4-oz apple looks like in the varieties of apples you like, or a 5-oz nectarine, or 3 1/2-oz kiwi.
- Cut large fruits in half, or count a whole piece of fruit as 2 servings or exchanges of fruit.

Fruit Juice

Portion control can be an even bigger challenge with fruit juice. One fruit exchange is about 4 ounces of juice. Yet 8 ounces is 1 serving according to the Nutrition Facts panel. If you gulp down 1 serving, you've actually drunk 2 fruit exchanges.

And juice often comes in 12- to 16-ounce containers. It's easy to chug down the whole thing and not realize you've had 3 to 4 fruit exchanges and a whole lot more calories than you wanted.

- Opt for pieces of fruit and not juice. With fruit you get fiber, and portion control is easier.
- Dilute a serving of fruit juice with carbonated mineral water or club soda. It's refreshing and gives you a larger drink with no more calories.

HOW MUCH JUICE?

Now fruit drinks that claim to contain juice must declare the total percentage of juice on the information panel, for example, "contains 10% real fruit juice."

In addition, FDA's regulation establishes criteria for naming juice beverages. For example, when the label of a juice beverage contains several types of juices and the fruit juice for which the beverage is named is present in minor amounts, the product's name must state that the beverage is flavored with that juice or declare the amount of the juice in a 5% range. For example: "raspberry-flavored juice blend" or "juice blend, 2 to 7% raspberry juice."

- Be aware that a fruit "drink" contains only 10% fruit juice. The rest is water sweetened with, usually, sugar or high-fructose corn syrup. In other words, it's a calorie-loaded, nutrition-lacking beverage. However, there are several fruit drinks on the market sweetened with a low-calorie sweetener (for example Oceanspray Lightstyles, Tropicana Twister Light). You can drink about 12 ounces and get only 60 calories, or the amount of calories in (though not the nutrition of) 1 fruit exchange.
- Avoid quenching your thirst with calorie- and carbohydrate-dense fruit juice. If it's a thirst quencher you need, try these low- to no-calorie ones instead:
  – Water (the best choice!)
  – Mineral water (carbonated or noncarbonated)
  – Flavored seltzer water (Check the label to make sure there are no calories.)
  – Flavored water made with low-calorie sweetener
  – Club soda
  – Diet tonic water
  – Diet soda
  – Powdered drink mix made with low-calorie sweetener
  – Lemonade made with low-calorie sweetener
  – Fruit drink beverage made with a low-calorie sweetener
  – Decaf tea (hot or iced)
  – Decaf coffee (hot or iced)

10 EXCELLENT SOURCES OF VITAMIN A

Food	Serving		% Daily Value
Cantaloupe	1/3	melon or	
	1	cup cubes	103%
Apricots, dried, fresh, canned, juice	1	serving	34–74%
Persimmon, Japanese	1		73%
Mango	1/2	fruit or	64%
	1/2	cup juice	
Passion fruit, juice (yellow)	1/2	cup	60%
Tangerine	2		31%
Mandarin oranges, canned	3/4	cup	31%
Plums, canned	1/2	cup	25%
Nectarine	1		20%
Peach	1	medium	18%

10 EXCELLENT SOURCES OF VITAMIN C

Food	Serving	% Daily Value
Guava	1	277%
Orange	1 (6 1/2 oz)	185%
Strawberries	1 1/4 cups	170%
Tangerine	2	123%
Cranberry juice, low-calorie	1 cup	116%
Cantaloupe	1/3 or 1 cup cubed	113%
Orange juice	1/2 cup	97%
Kiwi	1	95%
Grapefruit juice	1/2 cup	73%
Mango	1/2	48%

Q What has the most nutrition: fresh, canned, frozen, or dried fruit?

A It's so important to eat fruit that whatever form you manage to eat it in, that's a step in the right direction. If you find it difficult to keep enough fresh fruit around then use canned, frozen, or dried fruit.

Canned fruit can be kept on the shelf for a long time and it is always at the ready. The same can be said for dried fruit.

Frozen fruit is great to blend for fruit sauces or to use in a fruit shake. Make sure you buy just fruit and not fruit swimming in sugar syrup.

Q Isn't fruit just natural sugar that will raise blood glucose quickly?

A Yes, fruit is nearly 100% carbohydrate, and most of that is sugar. Yes, fruit will raise blood glucose, because that's what carbohydrates do. Don't avoid fruit as a way of keeping your blood glucose in control. Follow a healthy meal plan and then work with your health care provider and diabetes educator to find a medication plan that helps you keep your blood glucose in control.

Q Should I avoid eating fruit at breakfast and for snacks?

A Some people have been told to avoid eating fruit as a snack, or to avoid eating fruit at breakfast if they have a harder time controlling their blood glucose in the morning.

Don't avoid fruit without the evidence that fruit is a problem. Check your blood glucose about two hours after you eat fruit. The next day, skip the fruit and substitute another source of carbohydrate, or substitute another type of fruit. Does it make a difference?

If you find that fruit, or certain fruits, or certain forms of fruit skyrocket your blood glucose in the morning or at a snack, then opt for different foods and work fruits in at different times.

Also, check your portions of fruit. It might be that your blood glucose rises more than expected because the portions are too large.

FANCIFUL FRUITS

Why not try some of the more exotic fruits now and then? These specialty produce items are becoming more widely available each year and you will often find labels and flyers that accompany the fruits that are new to the market. All of the fruits below are great sources of vitamin C, potassium, and fiber and are virtually sodium-free.

Figs: Fresh figs (green Calimyrna or Black mission figs) are most available in the summer. Look for fruits with well-colored, unbroken skin; ripe figs will be plump, slightly soft to the touch, mildly fragrant. If necessary, ripen them in an open dish for a few days. To serve, simply cut off the stems and quarter the fruit to enjoy its soft, moist flesh filled with tiny crunchy seeds. A bit of lemon or orange juice enhances the flavor.

Pomegranate: This fruit holds pockets of flesh-covered edible seeds. Pomegranates are always sold ripe; choose heavy unbroken ones. Cut off the blossom end and score the skin to break the fruit in half, and pry out the seeds with your finger or a spoon. Be careful; the juice stains. Eat the morsels of fruit as a snack, use as a garnish, or juice and strain and use as a drink.

Papayas: Buy papayas that are at least half yellow, then ripen in a paper bag at room temperature until they are three quarters yellow-orange and yield to finger pressure. Serve seeded papaya halves as you would melon; fill them with seafood or salad. Add sliced papaya to green salads or fruit salads.

Pineapple: Although pineapples are not really that exotic these days, choosing one can be tricky. Once picked, a pineapple will not get sweeter, so be sure to choose a ripe one. Look for a plump, heavy, gold-tinged fruit with flexible, deep-green leaves. The ease with which a leaf can be pulled out is not a reliable guide to ripeness. Pass on pineapple with soft or dark spots, sunken eyes, or brown leaves. A ripe pineapple should be fragrant. To cut a pineapple follow these steps:

1. Grasp the leaves and twist them off the crown.

2. Cut a thin slice off the bottom and stand the pineapple upright. Using a large knife, pare off just enough skin to expose the "eyes."

3. Following the diagonal pattern of the "eyes," make wedged-shaped pattern cuts to remove them. Then quarter, slice, or dice the fruit as desired.

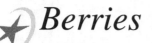 *Berries*

Mother Nature knew what she was doing when she arranged for the berries to be at their peak in summer. When the dog days hit and all you want to do is quietly turn the pages of a book, the fresh succulence of berries popping in your mouth will perhaps have you forget about the heat. Your body, however, will not forget the nutritional goodness you are giving it by eating berries. They are full of fiber, vitamin C, and phytochemicals that appear to deactivate potential carcinogens. And the many varieties of berries keep things interesting!

How to Buy and Store

Blueberry: Cultivated blueberries comprise the majority of the blueberries that reach the market and the season is generally from May to early October. Choose berries that are firm, uniform in size, indigo blue with a bit of a silver frost. Don't wash them until you're ready to use them. You can store them in the refrigerator for up to 5 days.

Blackberry: The highest in fiber of all the berries, with more fiber than a serving of bran cereal. Excellent source of vitamin C. The blacker the berry, the riper and sweeter the fruit. Fresh blackberries are best when eaten right away, but they can be kept refrigerated, preferably in a single layer (on a cookie sheet or on paper towels), for 1 to 2 days. Rinse just before you eat them.

Raspberry: Black, golden, and red raspberries are all excellent sources of fiber and vitamin C. Since raspberries are so fragile, do handle them with the utmost of care. Avoid shriveled or moldy berries. Store in a single layer in the refrigerator for 1 to 2 days.

Strawberry: The strawberry is a member of the rose family. The Romans believed the strawberry had therapeutic powers. Strawberries are the most hardy of the berries and can withstand shipping and storage. Choose brightly colored berries that still have their green tops intact. Berries don't ripen off the vine, so buy them full colored. Don't wash until ready to eat.

Out of Season?

Although it's tempting to purchase berries in the middle of the winter, they may not be tasty and will certainly be much more expensive than if you wait until they are in season. When berries or other fruits are out of season, buy frozen fruits with no sugar added.

How to Use Berries

Think of berries as more than just dessert. Fresh berries make a wonderful base for a sauce for chicken, beef, or seafood. Toss a few fresh raspberries into a main dish salad. Try a cooling berry soup as a first course. Use puréed berries as part of a salad dressing.

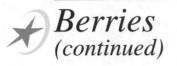

Berries
(continued)

When you are planning to use them as a dessert, berries are most divine in their natural form, eaten from a chilled bowl. However, there are ways to dress them up too:

- Layer berries in between nonfat plain yogurt spiked with vanilla extract. Top with toasted wheat germ or 1 tsp toasted walnuts.
- Slice some fat-free pound cake. Purée 1 cup raspberries in the blender with 2 tsp sugar and 1 Tbsp orange juice. Drizzle the raspberry purée over the cake.

- Beat 1/2 cup fat-free cream cheese with 2 tsp sugar. Add 1/4 tsp vanilla, almond, or orange extract. Add 1 Tbsp fat-free milk. Beat the mixture until light. Serve over 2 cups of berries.
- Top fat-free frozen yogurt with any of the berries. Add fat-free, sugar-free sundae syrup and you have the makings of a summer sundae party!

Citrus

Citrus fruits, including oranges, grapefruits, tangerines, and clementines, are terrific sources of vitamin C. Oranges are a good source of folate. Red and pink grapefruit contain lycopene, an antioxidant. When you eat whole citrus fruit (not just drink the juice), you get the fruit's bountiful fiber content as well.

How to Buy: Choose fruit that is heavy for its size with no mold or spongy spots. Grapefruit should be springy, yet firm when held in the palm and pressed.

How to Store: Citrus fruits should be kept in the refrigerator for no more than 2 weeks. Put in a plastic bag and store in the vegetable drawer.

Uses: Eat as fruit servings, add to salads and main dishes.

Blueberries with Almond Cream

Serving Size: about 1/2 cup, Total Servings: 4

This is an elegant way to dress up seasonal berries. You can also use the cream cheese topping to spread on homemade carrot or zucchini bread.

2 cups washed blueberries	**1** Tbsp powdered sugar
1/2 cup reduced-fat cream cheese (Neufchâtel)	**1/4** tsp almond extract
1 Tbsp fat-free milk	**2** Tbsp toasted sliced almonds

1 Divide the blueberries among four dessert dishes.

2 Using electric beaters, cream together the cream cheese, milk, and sugar until smooth. Add the extract and mix 10 seconds more. Fold in the almonds.

3 Serve the blueberries with a dollop of almond cream.

PREPARATION
10 minutes

Exchanges
1 Fruit
1 1/2 Fat

Calories	142
Calories from Fat	75
Total Fat	8 g
Saturated Fat	4 g
Cholesterol	20 mg
Sodium	127 mg
Carbohydrate	14 g
Dietary Fiber	2 g
Sugars	8 g
Protein	4 g

Blueberry Lemon Muffins

Serving Size: 1 muffin, Total Servings: 10 muffins

Perfect for tea time or a light snack, these muffins have a nice touch of lively lemon. The yogurt in the muffins takes the place of the oil and will give the muffin moisture. Be very careful to just gently fold the blueberries into the batter, so they can retain their plump, juicy appearance!

2 cups all-purpose flour	1 tsp lemon extract
1/4 cup brown sugar	1 egg
1 tsp baking powder	1 egg white
1/4 tsp baking soda	3/4 cup fresh blueberries
Pinch salt	Zest of 1 lemon
1 cup plain, nonfat yogurt	

1 Preheat the oven to 400°F. Lightly oil 10 standard-sized muffin cups or use nonstick bakeware.

2 In a large bowl, combine the flour, brown sugar, baking powder, baking soda, and salt. In a small bowl, beat together the yogurt, extract, egg, and egg white. Add the yogurt mixture to the flour mixture and mix until just combined. Fold in the blueberries and lemon zest.

3 Spoon the batter into the prepared muffin cups, two-thirds full. Bake for 15 minutes until a tester comes out clean and muffins are slightly browned.

4 Remove muffins from the oven. Let cool in the pan for 10 minutes. Turn out muffins and cool completely before storage.

PREPARATION
20 minutes

COOK
15 minutes

Exchanges
2 Starch

Calories 141
  Calories from Fat 7
Total Fat . . . . .1 g
  Saturated Fat . . . . .0 g
Cholesterol . . . . .22 mg
Sodium . . . . .109 mg
Carbohydrate . . . . .28 g
  Dietary Fiber . . . . .1 g
  Sugars . . . . .8 g
Protein . . . . .5 g

Strawberry-Peach Soup

Serving Size: about 1/2 cup, Total Servings: 4

Fruit soups are a refreshing way to start or end a meal. Their light sweetness will tease your palate for the meal to come or will finish your dining experience on a nice clean note. Use your imagination to create many fruit combinations. Other berries such as blueberries or raspberries may be used. Nectarines and fresh apricots are also nice.

1 cup fresh strawberries, hulled and washed	**3** Tbsp brown sugar
1 cup diced fresh peaches	**1/2** tsp lemon juice
1/2 cup plain, nonfat yogurt	**1** Tbsp minced fresh mint

1 In a food processor or blender, combine the strawberries and peaches. Blend until smooth.

2 Transfer the purée to a mixing bowl. Add the remaining ingredients, cover, and chill for 4–5 hours.

3 Pour into individual bowls and top with a dollop of low-fat sour cream or plain nonfat yogurt.

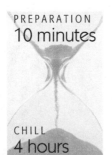

PREPARATION
10 minutes

CHILL
4 hours

Exchanges
1 1/2 Fruit

Calories 84
   Calories from Fat 2
Total Fat . . . . 0 g
   Saturated Fat . . . . 0 g
Cholesterol . . . . 1 mg
Sodium . . . . 28 mg
Carbohydrate . . . . 20 g
   Dietary Fiber . . . . 2 g
   Sugars . . . . 18 g
Protein . . . . 2 g

Strawberry Raspberry Almond Shake

Serving Size: about 3/4 cup, Total Servings: 4

Start the day off with this sprightly breakfast beverage! Change the extract to create many flavor sensations; try vanilla, coconut, lemon, orange, or even chocolate.

1 cup fresh strawberries, hulled and washed

1 cup fresh raspberries

1 cup fat-free milk

1/2 tsp almond extract

1/2 cup ice cubes

2 tsp sugar

1 Combine all ingredients in a blender and blend until smooth and creamy.

2 Pour into chilled glasses and serve.

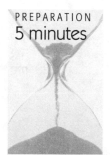

PREPARATION
5 minutes

Exchanges
1 Carbohydrate

Calories 56
   Calories from Fat 4
Total Fat . . . . 0 g
   Saturated Fat . . . . 0 g
Cholesterol . . . . 1 mg
Sodium . . . . 32 mg
Carbohydrate . . . . .11 g
   Dietary Fiber . . . . 3 g
   Sugars . . . . 8 g
Protein . . . . 3 g

Orange and Fennel Salad

Serving Size: about 1 cup, Total Servings: 6

A beautiful salad with so many complementing colors! Fennel has a slight licorice flavor that pairs well with tart oranges. Use fennel as you would use celery in fresh salads. We think fennel is much more exciting than celery. When buying fennel, look for plump-looking bulbs and bright green leaves.

Salad

- **4** cups torn romaine lettuce
- **1** cup torn radicchio leaves
- **3** large oranges, peeled and cut into slices crosswise, seeds removed
- **2** medium fennel bulbs, ends trimmed and thinly sliced

Dressing

- **3** Tbsp white wine vinegar
- **2** Tbsp olive oil
- **1** tsp honey
- **1** tsp chopped fennel leaves
- **1** clove garlic, minced
- **1/2** grated orange zest
- Fresh ground pepper and salt to taste

1 For the salad, combine the romaine and radicchio in a large bowl. Scatter fennel on top.

2 Whisk together all ingredients for the dressing. Pour over the salad and top with oranges.

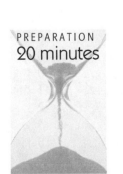

PREPARATION
20 minutes

Exchanges
1 Vegetable
1 Fruit   1 Fat

Calories 117
   Calories from Fat 40
Total Fat . . . . .4 g
   Saturated Fat . . . . .1 g
Cholesterol . . . . .0 mg
Sodium . . . . 45 mg
Carbohydrate . . . . 19 g
   Dietary Fiber . . . . 6 g
   Sugars . . . . .11 g
Protein . . . . .3 g

Grapefruit Combo Salad

Serving Size: 1 cup, Total Servings: 4

1 medium grapefruit, peeled and sectioned

1 medium orange, peeled and sectioned

1 medium red onion, sliced very thinly

1 small apple, diced

Dressing

1/4 cup orange juice

1 Tbsp sugar

2 Tbsp red wine vinegar

Salt and pepper to taste

1 Combine the grapefruit, orange, red onion, and apple in a salad bowl.

2 Whisk together the dressing ingredients. Pour over the salad, and chill salad for 1 hour.

3 Drain any excess liquid and serve over lettuce leaves if desired.

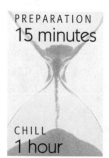

PREPARATION
15 minutes

CHILL
1 hour

Exchanges
1 1/2 Fruit

Calories 89
  Calories from Fat 3
Total Fat . . . . 0 g
  Saturated Fat . . . . 0 g
Cholesterol . . . . 0 mg
Sodium . . . . 1 mg
Carbohydrate . . . . 22 g
  Dietary Fiber . . . . 3 g
  Sugars . . . . 18 g
Protein . . . . 1 g

Mango

What would you guess an orange-colored fruit would feature? Yes, lots of vitamin A. A half a mango and you are more than halfway to your daily vitamin A goal. Mango is also an excellent source of vitamin C.

How to Buy: Mangoes are grown in Hawaii and California and are available in most parts of the country from May to September. Look for unblemished yellow skin blushed with red. Look for large mangoes so that there is a higher fruit-to-seed ratio. A ripe mango feels slightly soft to the touch and smells sweet.

How to Store: Underripe mangoes can be put in a paper bag and left to ripen at cool room temperature. Ripe man-

goes can be placed in a plastic bag and kept in the refrigerator for 5 days.

Uses: To slice a mango, make a lengthwise cut all around the large, flat pit, then make four vertical cuts on each side and strip the skin from each section. Slide a sharp knife under each section to cut the flesh off the pit. Eat sliced mango with a squeeze of lime. Toss into fruit salads, purée into smoothies, make into salsa, and toss into cold salads.

Cantaloupe

Cantaloupe is another orange-colored fruit packed with vitamin A. In addition, you get more vitamin C than the daily value and it nearly makes the grade as a good source of folate.

Kiwi

This plum-sized New Zealand native (grown in California as well) has a fuzzy brown skin. Its juicy lime-green flesh contains a sunburst of edible black seeds. The flavor has hints of strawberry and banana.

One medium kiwi provides potassium, and about 72 mg of vitamin C, more than the RDA for vitamin C for a day.

Look for plump fruits that yield to light pressure; ripen firm ones at home for a few days. Eat a halved kiwifruit with a spoon or peel and eat it whole. Use peeled sliced kiwi in salads, or purée the peeled fruit for a dessert sauce.

Lime Guacamole with Mango

Serving Size: 1 ounce chips with avocado and mango,
Total Servings: 4

This is a slimmed-down version of guacamole. It has a different twist with a lot more pizazz!

1	large avocado	**2**	tsp sugar
1	large mango	**1/2**	tsp minced jalapeño pepper
3	Tbsp fresh lime juice	**4**	oz baked corn tortilla chips

1 Cut the avocado in half lengthwise and pit. Scoop out the flesh. In a bowl, mash the avocado slightly with a fork.

2 Peel and cube the mango into 1/2-inch cubes and put into another bowl.

3 Add the lime juice, sugar, and jalapeño pepper divided equally between the avocado and mango.

4 To serve, put 2 tsp of mango on a chip. Add mashed avocado on top of the mango and eat!

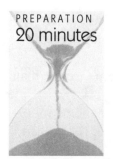

PREPARATION
20 minutes

Exchanges
1/2 Starch   1 Fruit
1 1/2 Fat

Calories 169
   Calories from Fat 73
Total Fat . . . . 8 g
   Saturated Fat . . . . 2 g
Cholesterol . . . . 0 mg
Sodium . . . . 46 mg
Carbohydrate . . . . 26 g
   Dietary Fiber . . . . 5 g
   Sugars . . . . .14 g
Protein . . . . 2 g

Pan-Seared Pork with Mango Salsa

Serving Size: 4 ounces, Total Servings: 4

For a pretty plate presentation, put the salsa on the bottom of a plate and place the pork in pinwheel fashion over the salsa. Garnish with fresh cilantro. You can also use chicken or shrimp for this recipe. You can use the mango mixture by itself, like a fruit salad.

1 lb boneless pork loin chops	1 medium mango, peeled and chopped
1/4 cup flour	1/2 cup diced canned pineapple
Salt and pepper	1/2 cup halved grapes
2 Tbsp olive oil	2 Tbsp lime juice
1/4 cup diced red onion	1 tsp sugar
1/4 cup diced red pepper	

1 On a plate or in a zippered plastic bag, combine the flour with salt and pepper. Coat the pork chops in the flour mixture. Shake off excess.

2 In a skillet over medium-high heat, heat the oil. Add the pork chops and cook until the pork chops are browned, about 7–9 minutes. Remove from the skillet and keep warm. Add the onion and red pepper to the skillet and sauté for 5 minutes.

3 Put the onion and pepper in a bowl. Add the mangoes, pineapple, grapes, lime juice, and sugar.

4 Serve the salsa with the pork.

PREPARATION
25 minutes

COOK
15 minutes

Exchanges
4 Lean Meat
1 1/2 Fruit

Calories 323
   Calories from Fat 121
Total Fat . . . . 13 g
   Saturated Fat . . . . 4 g
Cholesterol . . . . 70 mg
Sodium . . . . 166 mg
Carbohydrate . . . . 26 g
   Dietary Fiber . . . . 2 g
   Sugars . . . . 18 g
Protein . . . . 26 g

Mango Chicken Salad

Serving Size: about 3/4 cup, Total Servings: 4

We have been known to eat this salad every day! It's so much more interesting than plain chicken salad; the addition of mango and grapes adds color and a sweet foil for the meaty chicken. For a nice presentation, hollow out a whole pineapple or papaya and pile the mango chicken high for all to gaze upon.

2 cups cooked skinless, boneless chicken breasts, cubed into 2-inch pieces	**2** Tbsp minced scallions
	2 tsp minced parsley
1 large mango, peeled and cut into 1/2-inch cubes	**1** cup nonfat mayonnaise
	2 Tbsp low-fat sour cream
1/2 cup halved green grapes	**1** Tbsp fresh orange juice
1/2 cup sliced celery	**1/4** tsp ground ginger
1/4 cup minced red onion	Salt and pepper to taste

1 In a large salad bowl, combine the chicken, mango, grapes, red onion, scallions, and parsley.

2 In a small bowl, whisk together the mayonnaise, sour cream, orange juice, ginger, salt, and pepper.

3 Fold the dressing into the chicken salad. Cover and chill for 1 hour.

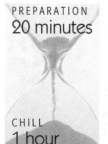

PREPARATION
20 minutes

CHILL
1 hour

Exchanges
1 Carbohydrate
3 Very Lean Meat
1 Fruit

Calories 239
    Calories from Fat 32
Total Fat . . . . 4 g
    Saturated Fat . . . . 1 g
Cholesterol . . . . 62 mg
Sodium . . . . 494 mg
Carbohydrate . . . . 27 g
    Dietary Fiber . . . . 2 g
    Sugars . . . . 20 g
Protein . . . . 24 g

Cool Melon Soup

Serving Size: about 3/4 cup, Total Servings: 4

Another clever way to get your fruit is to make pretty-as-a picture fruit soups. Although the Grand Marnier is optional, this small bit of alcohol will bring out the orange flavor in the orange juice and pairs well with the cantaloupe. Make sure to chill this soup thoroughly so the flavors have a chance to blend. Fruit soups are best when served nice and cold. Consider hollowing out cantaloupe halves and use as a bowl for the soup.

2 cups chopped cantaloupe

1/4 cup fresh orange juice

1 cup plain nonfat yogurt

2 tsp sugar

2 tsp minced mint

1 tsp Grand Marnier (optional)

Garnish: mint sprigs

1 In a blender, combine 1 cup of the cantaloupe with the remaining ingredients and blend until smooth, about 1 minute.

2 Fold in the remaining cantaloupe and pour into a container and chill for at least 2 hours. Serve in soup bowls garnished with mint sprigs.

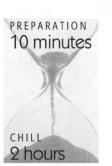

PREPARATION
10 minutes

CHILL
2 hours

Exchanges
1 Carbohydrate

Calories 73
   Calories from Fat 2
Total Fat . . . . 0 g
   Saturated Fat . . . . 0 g
Cholesterol . . . . 1 mg
Sodium . . . . 55 mg
Carbohydrate . . . . 15 g
   Dietary Fiber . . . . 1 g
   Sugars . . . . 14 g
Protein . . . . 4 g

Orange and Kiwi Salad

Serving Size: 1 cup, Total Servings: 6

Boost the vitamin C content (and the color) of your salad with the addition of kiwis and oranges. Choose dark lettuces over iceberg lettuce. Dark lettuces usually have more vitamin C and fiber than light-colored ones do.

3/4 lb romaine lettuce
(about 1 small head)

3 small kiwi fruits, peeled and sliced into 1/4-inch rounds

2 oranges, peeled and sliced into 1/2-inch rounds

3 Tbsp apple cider or champagne vinegar

1 tsp lemon juice
Salt and pepper to taste

2 Tbsp walnut oil or olive oil

1 small red onion, sliced into rings

1 Wash the lettuce and tear into bite-sized pieces. Put the lettuce on a serving platter. Top the lettuce with the kiwis and oranges placed in a circular pattern.

2 Combine the vinegar, lemon juice, pepper, salt, and oil in a small bowl. Whisk until blended. Drizzle the dressing over the salad.

3 Top the salad with red onion rings.

PREPARATION
20 minutes

Exchanges
1 Fruit
1 Fat

Calories 103
   Calories from Fat 45
Total Fat . . . . .5 g
   Saturated Fat . . . . .0 g
Cholesterol . . . . .0 mg
Sodium . . . . .7 mg
Carbohydrate . . . . .14 g
   Dietary Fiber . . . . .4 g
   Sugars . . . . .10 g
Protein . . . . .2 g

Minted Kiwi Salad

Serving Size: about 1 cup, Total Servings: 4

This is more than just fruit salad, it's a fruit presentation. You can be proud to serve this at any occasion. By placing the fruit in rows and serving an elegant sauce on the side, fruit gets elevated from lowly status to one of great beauty. The fresh mint provides a cool complement to the slight tangy taste of the strawberries and oranges.

2 kiwi fruits, peeled and sliced into 1/4-inch thick rounds

1 banana, sliced into 1/2-inch thick rounds

1 cup sliced strawberries

1 orange, sectioned

Dressing

1 cup nonfat, sugar-free vanilla yogurt

2 Tbsp fresh minced mint

1/2 tsp cinnamon

1 On a platter, arrange the kiwi, banana, strawberries, and orange in rows.

2 Combine the dressing ingredients. Serve the dressing with the fruit.

PREPARATION
20 minutes

Exchanges
1 1/2 Fruit

Calories 113
  Calories from Fat 5
Total Fat . . . . .1 g
  Saturated Fat . . . . .0 g
Cholesterol . . . . .1 mg
Sodium . . . . .38 mg
Carbohydrate . . . . .26 g
  Dietary Fiber . . . . .4 g
  Sugars . . . . .18 g
Protein . . . . .3 g

Along with the crisp mornings and the kaleidoscope of falling leaves, apples take center stage on our fall dining tables. Apples are a good source of fiber and vitamins A and C. It's no wonder they keep the doc at bay.

Apples have been cultivated for at least 3,000 years. There are so many varieties, it can get confusing which to use for what purpose. Let's look at some of the most common varieties.

Braeburn: Their texture is very firm. Good for salads, pies, and baking. Best season is October through July.

Criterion: Their flavor is best described as sweet and complex. A personal favorite. Very good for salads and pies and good for baking. Best season is from October through March.

Elstar: Their texture is firm, their flavor tart-sweet. Very good for salads and baking, good for pies. Their season is September to March.

Fuji: Their texture is crisp, flavor sweet-spicy. Excellent for salads. Good for pies and baking. Available year-round.

Gala: Their texture is sweet and crisp. Very good for salads. Good for pies and baking. Best season is August through March.

Golden Delicious: Tender texture, sweet flavor. Very good for salads, excellent for pies and baking. Available year-round.

Granny Smith: Crisp and tart. Very good for salads, pies, and baking. Available year-round.

Jonagold: Crisp and sweet-tart. Very good for salads, pies, and baking. Best season is from September to April.

Newtown-Pippin: Firm texture, slightly tart flavor. Very good for salads and baking, excellent for pies. Best season is from September to June.

Red Delicious: Sweet and crisp. Excellent for salads and eating out of hand. Fair for pies; not really good for baking. Available year-round.

Rome Beauty: Firm texture, slightly tart. Good for salads. Very good for pies and excellent for baking. The best season is September to July.

Winesap: Their texture firm, their flavor slightly tart and spicy. Excellent for salads, good for pies and baking. Best season is from October through April.

APPLE OF MY EYE

Whatever the variety, look for apples that are firm and have a fresh fragrance. Store your apples in a cool, dark place. They do well in a plastic bag stored in the refrigerator. Apples emit ethylene, a gas that hastens ripening; putting an apple in a bag with unripe bananas will result in ripe bananas. Watch out though: Fruits in a bowl near apples may become overripe.

Uses

Apples are so versatile. Besides just crunching on a juicy, ripe apple here are some enticing ideas for this fabulous fruit:

- Serve apple wedges with cubes of low-fat cheese. Always a winning combination, the duo will provide more vitamins and minerals than having a hunk of chocolate cake for dessert.
- Halved and cored apples make natural boats for cottage cheese or salad combinations.
- To accompany a chicken or lean-meat dinner, slice an apple and sprinkle with orange juice and nutmeg and then bake at 350°F for 10-15 minutes until soft.
- Roasted apples on the barbecue is a dream dessert! For each apple (use Granny Smith), slice and core. Put each apple on a sheet of foil.

Sprinkle the apple very lightly with 1 tsp brown sugar and 1 tsp lemon juice. Add a sprinkle of cinnamon and dot with 1 tsp low-calorie margarine. Fold up the foil to make a packet. Place the packet over medium coals and cook for 20 minutes until the apple is soft. Carefully remove from the grill and open the packet.

- Sliced apples with just a smear of low-fat peanut butter is a great after-school, after-work healthy snack.
- Add diced apples to hot oatmeal as it cooks. The apple juice will naturally sweeten the oatmeal; no need for sugar!

Apple Sandwiches

Serving Size: 1 sandwich, Total Servings: 4

If you have trouble thinking of ways to eat more fruit, add it to your meals as part of the main or side dish. Here, the apple adds a pleasant sweetness to the slightly smoky and salty taste of lean ham. Use lean diced turkey or chicken in place of the ham if desired.

1 apple, unpeeled and finely chopped (use any type of apple you like)

4 oz lean ham, diced

1/4 cup finely diced celery

1/3 cup low-fat mayonnaise

1 tsp lemon juice
Salt and pepper to taste

4 butter lettuce leaves

8 thin slices whole-wheat bread

1 In a medium sized bowl, combine the apple, ham, celery, mayonnaise, lemon juice, salt, and pepper. Mix well.

2 Spread the apple-ham mixture on 4 slices of whole wheat bread. Add lettuce leaf. Top with remaining bread slice.

PREPARATION
15 minutes

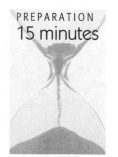

Exchanges
1 Starch
1 Lean Meat
1 Fruit

Calories 180
  Calories from Fat 32
Total Fat . . . . 4 g
  Saturated Fat . . . . 0 g
Cholesterol . . . . .16 mg
Sodium . . . . 810 mg
Carbohydrate . . . . 29 g
  Dietary Fiber . . . . 6 g
  Sugars . . . . .10 g
Protein . . . . .12 g

Red Cherry Frozen Yogurt Sundae

Serving Size: 1 sundae, Total Servings: 4

Sour cherries are smaller and softer than sweet cherries. While too tart to eat raw, sour cherries are best for pie making and preserves. The cherry season is short in most parts of the country, but fortunately canned sour cherries are available. This recipe adds a little zip to frozen yogurt. Try the sauce over slices of low-fat, low-sugar cakes too.

1/3 cup sugar

1 Tbsp cornstarch or arrowroot

1 (16-oz) can sour cherries, drained, reserve 1/2 cup of liquid

1/4 tsp vanilla

2 cups low-fat frozen vanilla yogurt

1 In a saucepan over low, combine the sugar and cornstarch. Stir well to keep the cornstarch from clumping and cook for 1 minute.

2 Add the reserved juice from the cherries to the sugar-cornstarch mixture. Cook over low heat, stirring constantly until thick and clear, about 2–3 minutes. Add the cherries and cook for 10 minutes, stirring occasionally. Add the extract and remove the cherries from the heat.

3 Scoop the yogurt into 4 serving dishes. Pour 1/2 cup of the cherries over each serving of yogurt.

PREPARATION
5 minutes

COOK
15 minutes

Exchanges
3 Carbohydrate

Calories 215
    Calories from Fat 14
Total Fat . . . . .2 g
    Saturated Fat . . . . .1 g
Cholesterol . . . . .8 mg
Sodium . . . . .47 mg
Carbohydrate . . . . .48 g
    Dietary Fiber . . . . .2 g
    Sugars . . . . .35 g
Protein . . . . .4 g

Red Grape and Turkey Salad

Serving Size: about 4 ounces, Total Servings: 4

Got leftover turkey from your holiday meal? Pair turkey with seasonal red grapes, toss in a few walnuts and celery for crunch, and you have a nice winter turkey salad. Of course, you can substitute chicken for the turkey. Use green or purple grapes if red aren't available. It's best to use seedless grapes.

- **2** tsp olive oil
- **1** lb boneless, skinless turkey filets, cut into 2-inch cubes (or 2 cups cooked turkey)
- **1** cup halved red grapes
- **1/2** cup diced celery
- **1/4** cup toasted walnuts

- **3/4** cup low-fat mayonnaise
- **1** Tbsp fresh lemon juice
- **1** tsp lemon zest
- **1** tsp Dijon mustard
  Salt and pepper to taste

1 In a medium skillet over medium-high heat, heat the oil. Add the turkey and sauté for 5-6 minutes until turkey is cooked through. Set aside.

2 In a medium bowl, combine the red grapes, celery, and walnuts. Add the turkey to the bowl.

3 In a small bowl, whisk the mayonnaise with the lemon juice, lemon zest, Dijon mustard, salt, and pepper. Fold dressing into turkey grape salad. Refrigerate, covered, for 1/2 hour.

PREPARATION
20 minutes

COOK
6 minutes

Exchanges
1 1/2 Carbohydrate
3 Lean Meat   1/2 Fat

Calories 311
    Calories from Fat 125
Total Fat . . . . .14 g
    Saturated Fat . . . . .0 g
Cholesterol . . . . .63 mg
Sodium . . . . .523 mg
Carbohydrate . . . . .22 g
    Dietary Fiber . . . . .1 g
    Sugars . . . . .15 g
Protein . . . . .25 g

Pears Baked with White Wine

Serving Size: 1/2 pear, Total Servings: 4

Sometimes pears can be a little dry and hard. For a softer, creamier pear, try baking them. Baking in white wine renders a delicious sauce that can be poured over the pears at serving time. This is a nice change from baked apples.

2 large pears, halved and cored	**1/2** tsp cinnamon
1 cup dry white wine	**1** Tbsp lemon juice
1 Tbsp honey	

1 Preheat the oven to 375°F. Put the pears cut side down in a baking dish. Pour the white wine, honey, cinnamon, and lemon juice over the pears. Bake uncovered for 25–30 minutes until pears are soft.

2 Remove the pears from the pan and spoon over any accumulated juices.

PREPARATION
5 minutes

COOK
30 minutes

Exchanges
1 1/2 Fruit

Calories 93
  Calories from Fat 4
Total Fat . . . . 0 g
  Saturated Fat . . . . 0 g
Cholesterol . . . . 0 mg
Sodium . . . . 2 mg
Carbohydrate . . . . 21 g
  Dietary Fiber . . . . 3 g
  Sugars . . . . 17 g
Protein . . . . 0 g

Island Sundaes

Serving Size: 1/2 cup, Total Servings: 4

Another way to dress up frozen yogurt is to add a pineapple flavor. Canned pineapple is actually one of the fruits we like canned. As with the Red Cherry Sundaes, use this pineapple sauce to top low-fat low-sugar cakes.

1 cup canned pineapple chunks packed in its own juice, drained; reserve 1/2 cup juice	**2** tsp cornstarch or arrowroot
	1 tsp butter
1 Tbsp brown sugar	**2** cups fat-free frozen vanilla yogurt

1 Combine the reserved pineapple juice with the brown sugar and cornstarch in a medium saucepan. Cook over medium heat, stirring constantly until thick, about 5 minutes.

2 Add the butter and pineapple chunks and cook for 1–2 minutes.

3 Spoon the pineapple sauce over the frozen yogurt and serve immediately.

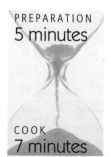

PREPARATION
5 minutes

COOK
7 minutes

Exchanges
2 1/2 Carbohydrate

Calories 171
　Calories from Fat 9
Total Fat . . . . 1 g
　Saturated Fat . . . . 1 g
Cholesterol . . . . 2 mg
Sodium . . . . 77 mg
Carbohydrate . . . . 37 g
　Dietary Fiber . . . . 1 g
　Sugars . . . . 20 g
Protein . . . . 4 g

	Exchange/ Serving	Calories	Carbohydrate (g)	Fiber (g)
Fruit, fresh				
Apple, unpeeled, small	1 (4 oz)	63	16	3
Apricots	4	68	16	3
Banana, small	1 (4 oz)	64	16	2
Blackberries	3/4 cup	56	14	5
Blueberries	3/4 cup	61	15	3
Cantaloupe	1 cup	56	13	1
Cherries, sweet	12 (3 oz)	59	14	2
Cranberries	1 cup	47	12	4
Figs, large	1 1/2	71	18	3
Grapefruit	1/2	51	13	2
Grapes, seedless	17	60	15	1
Honeydew melon	1 cup	59	16	1
Kiwi	1	56	14	3
Mango	1/2 cup	68	18	2
Nectarine	1	67	16	2
Orange	1 (6 1/2 oz)	62	15	3
Papaya	1 cup	55	14	3
Peach, medium	1 (6 oz)	57	15	3
Pear, large	1/2 (4 oz)	59	15	2
Pineapple	3/4 cup	57	14	1
Plums, small	2 (5 oz)	73	17	2
Raspberries, black, red	1 cup	60	14	8
Rhubarb	2 cups	52	11	4
Strawberries	1 1/4 cups	56	13	4
Tangerine, small	2 (8 oz)	74	19	3
Watermelon, cubed	1 1/4 cups	64	14	1
Fruit, canned or jarred, with some juice				
Applesauce, unsweetened	1/2 cup	52	14	2
Apricots	1/2 cup	60	15	2
Cherries, sweet, juice packed	1/2 cup	68	17	1
Cranberry sauce	1/4 cup	86	22	1

(continued)

Fruit

	Exchange/ Serving	Calories	Carbohydrate (g)	Fiber (g)
Fruit, canned or jarred, with some juice (cont'd)				
Fruit cocktail, juice packed	1/2 cup	57	15	1
Fruit cocktail	1/2 cup	55	14	1
Grapefruit, juice packed	3/4 cup	69	17	1
Mandarin oranges	3/4 cup	69	18	1
Peaches, juice packed	1/2 cup	55	14	1
Pears, juice packed	1/2 cup	62	16	3
Pineapple, juice packed	1/2 cup	74	20	1
Plums, juice packed	1/2 cup	73	19	1
Pumpkin, solid packed	3/4 cup	59	15	6
Fruit, dried				
Apples, rings	4	63	17	2
Apricots, halves	8	66	17	3
Dates	3	68	18	2
Figs	1 1/2	71	18	3
Fruit snacks, chewy, roll	1	78	18	1
Prunes, uncooked	3	60	16	2
Raisins, dark, seedless	2 Tbsp	54	14	1
Fruit, frozen unsweetened				
Blackberries	3/4 cup	73	18	6
Blueberries	3/4 cup	58	14	3
Melon balls	1 cup	57	14	1
Raspberries	1/2 cup	61	15	6
Strawberries	1 1/4 cups	65	17	4
Fruit juices				
Apple juice/cider	1/2 cup	58	15	0
Apricot nectar	1/2 cup	70	17	0
Cranapple juice cocktail	1/3 cup	53	13	0
Cranberry juice cocktail	1/3 cup	48	12	0
Fruit juice bars, 100% juice	1	75	19	0
Grape juice	1/3 cup	51	13	0
Orange juice, fresh	1/2 cup	56	13	0
Orange juice, from frozen	1/2 cup	56	13	0
Pineapple juice, canned	1/2 cup	70	17	0
Prune juice	1/3 cup	60	15	1

FOCUS ON Fiber

There are two types of dietary fiber, and each has health benefits.

Insoluble Fibers

Cellulose, hemicellulose, and lignin are insoluble fibers. Whole grain cereals and breads contain insoluble fiber.

Insoluble fiber also keeps bowel movements softer and bulkier, which promotes regularity and may prevent hemorrhoids and diverticulosis. High-fiber diets have been associated with lower risks of colon and rectal cancer.

Soluble Fiber

Soluble fiber is thick and gummy. Gums, mucilages, and pectin are examples of soluble fiber. Beans, peas, oats, and barley have soluble fiber.

A high intake of soluble fiber can lower blood cholesterol a small amount.

Fit in Fiber

A healthy intake of fiber is 20 to 35 grams a day from a variety of foods. Most Americans get only 11 to 13 grams a day. You'll likely get the recommended amount of fiber if most of your food choices come from starches, vegetables, and fruit, and you make the higher-fiber choices.

10 BEST SOURCES OF FIBER IN THE STARCH GROUP

Food	Serving	Fiber (g)
Bran cereal (for example: All Bran, 100% Bran, Bran Buds, Fiber One)	1/2 cup	10–18
Acorn squash, boiled or baked	1 cup	7–11
Butternut squash	1 cup	6–7
Dried beans, peas, lentils	1/2 cup	5–8
Bran Flake cereals	3/4 cup	4–6
Rye wafer cracker	4	5
Peas, green, frozen, boiled	1/2 cup	5
Bulgur, cooked	1/2 cup	4
Corn, cooked	1/2 cup, 1 (5-oz) cob	4
Air popped popcorn	3 cups	4

10 BEST SOURCES OF FIBER IN THE VEGETABLE GROUP

Food	Serving	Fiber (g)
Brussels sprouts, cooked	1/2 cup	4
Artichoke	1/2	3
Spinach, cooked	1/2 cup	3
Broccoli, cooked	1/2 cup	3
Greens, cooked	1/2 cup	3
Jicama, raw	1/2 cup	3
Pea pods/snow peas, cooked	1/2 cup	2
Okra, cooked	1/2 cup	2
Green beans, cooked	1/2 cup	2
Tomato products	1 serving	2

10 BEST SOURCES OF FIBER IN THE FRUIT GROUP

Food	Serving	Fiber (g)
Red raspberries	1 cup	5
Blackberries	3/4 cup	5
Blueberries	3/4 cup	4
Strawberries	1 1/4 cups	3
Prunes	3	3
Dried apricots	8 halves	3
Dried figs	1 1/2	3
Apple	1 small	3
Orange	1 small	2
Pear	1/2 large fresh	2

Tips to Eat More Fiber

Dry Cereals

* Look for dry cereals that contain "whole grain." Look for a health claim about whole grains on cereal boxes. As of 1999, manufacturers are allowed to put a health claim about the benefit of whole grains in relation to heart disease.

* Buy dry cereals that contain at least 3 grams of dietary fiber per serving.

* Buy a dry cereal that contains at least 7 grams of dietary fiber, such as All Bran, Bran Buds, Bran Flakes, or Grape Nut nuggets. Mix a small amount of that into a lower-fiber cereal if you don't like the taste of the high-fiber cereal alone.

* Sprinkle a tablespoon of toasted wheat germ or ground flax seed on your cereal for an added gram of fiber.

Hot Cereals

* Buy hot cereals that contain at least 3 grams of dietary fiber per serving, such as Maypo, Wheatena, Oatbran, or oatmeal.

* Sprinkle a tablespoon of toasted wheat germ or ground flax seed on your hot cereal for an added gram of fiber (as well as other important nutrients), or mix in some All Bran or Grape Nuts.

Crackers

* Buy crackers that contain at least 2 grams of dietary fiber per serving.

* Look for whole-grain crackers.

Add Fiber to Meals and Snacks

* Work high-fiber foods—bulgur, wheat germ, ground flax seed, All Bran or Grape Nuts, and seeds—into meat loaf, stuffing, and grain dishes.

* Incorporate a few nuts into salads, casseroles, and desserts. (Do remember that nuts are high in fat.)

* Choose whole-wheat pasta, brown rice, whole-wheat couscous, and the whole-grain alternative for as many foods as possible.

* When you prepare brown rice, other whole-grain starches, or beans, make extra and toss into salads, casseroles, or soups.

* Microwave some frozen peas or corn and toss a handful on salads.

* Incorporate all types of beans into your meal planning. Try them in soups, on salads, and in casseroles.

Here's how one fiber-rich day looks:

BREAKFAST

Food	Amount	Fiber (g)	Calories
Bran Flakes	1/2 cup	3	63
All Bran	1/4 cup	5	82
Wheat germ	1 Tbsp	1	27
Fat-free milk	1 cup	0	86
Blueberries	3/4 cup	4	61

LUNCH

Food	Amount	Fiber (g)	Calories
Wheat bread	2 slices	6	179
Romaine lettuce	2 leaves	0	1
Chicken breast	2 oz	0	112
Popcorn	3 cups popped	3	90
Apple with skin	1 small	3	81
Oatmeal raisin cookies	2 small	1	120

DINNER

Food	Amount	Fiber (g)	Calories
Marinated flank steak	4 oz, cooked	0	220
Baked potato with skin	1 medium	3	132
Sour cream, light	1 Tbsp	0	20
Broccoli, cooked	1/2 cup	2	22
Mixed green salad	1 cup	1	9
Soy nuts, dry (to top salad)	1 Tbsp	1	48
Italian dressing	1 Tbsp	0	45

SNACK

Food	Amount	Fiber (g)	Calories
Low-fat yogurt	1 cup	0	137
Raisins	2 Tbsp	1	62
Low-fat granola	2 Tbsp	1	45
Daily Totals:		35	1600

Check the Food Label

Fat-free Refried Beans

Nutrition Facts
Serving Size: 1/2 cup (124 g)
Servings per Container: About 3 1/2

	AMOUNT PER SERVING
Calories	100
Calories from Fat	0

	% DAILY VALUE
Total Fat 0 g	0%
Cholesterol 0 mg	0%
Sodium 480 mg	20%
Total Carbohydrate 18 g	6%
Dietary Fiber 6 g	24%
Sugars 1 g	0%
Protein 6 g	0%

Food labels can help you pick higher-fiber foods.

The amount of dietary fiber is required information on the Nutrition Facts panel on most foods. Dietary fiber is indented under Total Carbohydrate.

Some manufacturers list the amount of soluble or insoluble fiber in their products if they have something to brag about or if they have made a nutrition claim about the product's fiber content.

In addition, the FDA now allows food manufacturers to place a health claim on fruits, vegetables, and grain products that contain fiber, particularly soluble fiber. The health claim will say something about lowering the risk of coronary heart disease or some cancers.

Fiber Term	Means
High or excellent source	5 grams or more of fiber per serving
Good source	2.5 to 4.9 grams per serving
More, enriched, or added	at least 2.5 grams per serving

Adjusting Insulin for Fiber

If you're on a multiple daily injection insulin regimen (you take insulin 3 to 4 times a day) or you use an insulin pump, you may need to adjust the amount of rapid-acting insulin you take before a high-fiber meal.

If the food or meal you plan to eat has 5 or more grams of fiber, subtract the grams of fiber from the total grams of carbohydrate in the meal. Then use your usual carbohydrate-to-insulin ratio. For example, say you choose the following breakfast:

Food	Carbohydrate (g)	Fiber (g)
3/4 cup high-fiber cereals	32	6
1 cup of fat-free milk	12	0
1 cup sliced strawberries	15	2
One slice whole-grain bread	17	3
Totals	76	11

The 11 grams of dietary fiber won't be digested and won't raise your blood sugar level. Therefore, base your dose of rapid-acting insulin on 65 grams of carbohydrate (76 − 11 = 65).

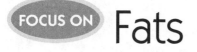

FOCUS ON Fats

In the top half of the food pyramid are the milk, meat, and fat groups. Except for the fat-free versions (fat-free milk), foods in these groups contain fat—some healthy and some not—so healthy.

The kind of fats you eat affects your blood lipid levels, which in turn affects your risk for having a heart attack.

People with either type 1 or type 2 diabetes are at increased risk of developing heart disease compared with the general population. People who have type 2 diabetes have two to four times the risk of developing heart disease as people who don't have diabetes. Abnormal blood lipid levels are a risk factor for heart disease. Therefore, bringing blood lipid levels into the healthy ranges is particularly important for people with diabetes.

Four measures of lipids in blood that you've probably heard of are:

HDL ("good") cholesterol

High-density lipoproteins (HDL) carry cholesterol to the liver, and the liver disposes of it. (HDL cholesterol is not in food, it's only in your blood.) A low HDL level is a risk factor for heart disease.

LDL ("bad") cholesterol

Low-density lipoproteins (LDL) carry cholesterol through the bloodstream and lay down fatty deposits or "plaque" on artery walls. (LDL cholesterol is not in food, it's only in your blood.) A high LDL level is a risk factor for heart disease.

Triglycerides

Triglycerides are your body's storage form of fat. A high blood triglyceride level is a risk factor for heart disease. Often, when blood glucose levels are high, the triglyceride level is high as well. When blood glucose is brought under control, triglyceride levels may decrease as well. The most common pattern of abnormal blood fats in type 2 diabetes is a high triglyceride level and a low HDL level.

Total cholesterol

Cholesterol travels in the bloodstream as a component of lipoproteins in both HDL cholesterol and

LDL cholesterol. Total cholesterol used to be considered the only blood lipid number to focus on to estimate the risk of heart disease. Today it's thought that additional indicators of cardiovascular health are the HDL, LDL, and triglyceride levels.

Blood Lipid Goals for People with Diabetes

(These are slightly different than for the general population.)

HDL	Greater than 45 mg/dl for men, Greater than 55 mg/dl for women
LDL	Less than or equal to 100 mg/dl
Triglycerides	Less than or equal to 200 mg/dl
Total cholesterol	Less than or equal to 200 mg/dl

Fat in Food

There are three broad categories of fat in food, and they affect blood lipid levels differently.

The Really Good Fats: Monounsaturated

Monounsaturated fats raise the HDL cholesterol and lower LDL cholesterol. That's why monounsaturated fats are known as good fats. The best sources of monounsaturated fats are canola, olive, and peanut oil; and olives, almonds, avocado, and peanuts.

The Pretty Good Fats: Polyunsaturated

On the positive, polyunsaturated fats help lower blood cholesterol, but on the negative side, they also lower HDLs. That's the wrong way for HDLs to go! So polyunsaturated fats aren't as good as monounsaturated fats, but they're far better than saturated fats.

Certain types of polyunsaturated fats are particularly good: omega-3 fats. Some research shows that omega-3 fats might help reduce heart disease by preventing blood platelets from clotting and sticking to the walls of arteries. Some research has related a large intake of omega-3 fats to a reduction in some cancers.

Plant sources of omega-3 fats are flax seeds and flax-seed oil, canola and walnut oil, and walnuts. Animal sources are fatty fish such as salmon, mackerel, sardines, herring. A number of these foods are among our Nutrition Superstars.

Saturated Fat

Saturated fat raises blood cholesterol (both HDL and LDL). Saturated fat is found mainly in fat from animal products: meats, fish, poultry, whole milk, full-fat cheeses and dairy foods, and butter. Non-animal sources of saturated fat are coconut oil, palm, and palm-kernel oil.

Cholesterol

Cholesterol is not fat, but a fat-like substance that raises blood cholesterol.

Cholesterol is found only in animal products.

It used to be thought that cholesterol in food had the biggest effect on blood cholesterol. Today we realize that saturated fat has the greatest effect on blood cholesterol. About 70% of cholesterol is manufactured by the liver, and about 30% is consumed in foods.

What Kind, How Much?

Two recommendations about the amount of fat you eat apply to most people:

* Limit saturated fat to less than 10% of your total calories.

* Consume no more than 300 mg cholesterol daily.

Other recommendations depend on your blood lipid levels and health goals. For example, if your LDL cholesterol is too high, you may be advised to lower your saturated fat intake to 7% of total calories and limit your cholesterol intake to 200 mg per day. If you want to lose weight, you may want to reduce calories from fat.

How Many Grams?

Here's how to figure out how much total fat and the other types of fats you need. We'll use about a 1,500-calorie intake as an example:

Take total number of calories: 1500
Multiply by 30%: 1500 x 0.30 = 450 calories from fat
Divide calories from fat by 9 (9 calories per gram of fat): 450 / 9 = 50 grams of fat

For the number of grams of saturated and polyunsaturated fat to stay under 10%:
1500 x 0.10 = 150 calories
150 / 9 = 17 grams

For the grams of monounsaturated fat to increase to at least 10% to 15%:
1500 x 0.10 and 0.15 = 150 and 225 calories
150 / 9 and 225 / 9 = 17 to 25 grams

How Many Grams to Eat?

This chart tells how many grams of fat to eat if you want to get 20%, 30%, or 40% of your calories as total fat for various calorie ranges. Don't forget to split total fat into the categories of fat according to your blood fat levels and your diabetes nutrition goals.

Calorie level	About 1200	About 1400	About 1600	About 1800	About 2200	About 2800
Fat grams (20%)	27	31	36	40	49	62
Fat grams (30%)	40	47	53	60	73	93
Fat grams (40%)	53	62	71	80	98	124

Nutrition Facts for Fats

Nutrition Facts labels have a lot of information about fat, and that can help you keep your meal plan on track.

Penne Pasta with Sun-Dried Tomatoes [a frozen entrée]

Nutrition Facts

Serving Size: 1 package
Servings per Container: 1

	AMOUNT PER SERVING
Calories	300
① **Calories from Fat**	70

	% DAILY VALUE
② **Total Fat** 8 g	12%
③ **Saturated Fat** 4 g	20%
Polyunsaturated Fat 1.5 g	
Monounsaturated Fat 2.5 g	
④ **Cholesterol** 15 mg	5%
Sodium 560 mg	23%
Total Carbohydrate 43 g	14%
Dietary Fiber 3 g	12%
Protein 11 g	.0%

① Calories from Fat

You can use this number to do a quick estimate of percent calories from fat. In your head, divide fat calories by total calories. In this example, it comes out to about 24%. Just calculate with round numbers, you'll get close enough.

Estimating the percent calories from fat can help reveal hidden fat. For example, many people think of crackers as a low-fat snack. A glance at the Nutrition Facts for one brand reveals that a serving is 70 calories from fat, and 150 calories total. That's nearly 50% fat!

But relying only on percent calories from fat can send you off in the wrong direction. Say your goal is to eat less than 30% of total calories as fat per day. A low-calorie Italian dressing you check might have 80% of calories from fat. Does that mean you shouldn't buy the salad dressing because it's over 30% fat? No. Remember, the 30% is per day, not per food. Another food you eat the same day, say canned peaches, may have 0 calories from fat.

In addition, percent calories from fat can sometimes be misleading. If you put a drop of oil in a glass of water, 100% of the calories are from fat, because water has no calories. But a drop is very little fat in grams. A serving of the low-calorie Italian salad dressing (2 Tbsp) has 3 grams of fat. Some of its other ingredients— water and vinegar—have no calories, so fat accounts for a big percent of the calories.

Therefore, you'll want to check out the total fat grams in a food to see if it fits in your meal plan.

② Total Fat Grams

Think about your daily goal for fat grams. Let's say it's 60 grams.

Relate that number to the total number of fat grams in the food. Think about the type of food it is: a meal, a beverage, a snack, or side dish. This meal has 8 grams of fat for a main course. That's low. However, if there are 8 grams of fat in a serving of crackers, you might want to move to a lower-fat or fat-free variety.

③ Grams of Saturated, Polyunsaturated, and Monounsaturated Fat

Saturated fat is on almost every label. The other fats must be noted if a manufacturer makes a claim about a product; otherwise they're optional. Remember you want to keep saturated fat down and monounsaturated fats up.

④ Cholesterol

The Nutrition Facts show cholesterol as amount (mg) and as a percent Daily Value, which is 300 mg. If your goal is 300 mg or less, as it is for most people, you can use the percent Daily Value no matter what your calorie range.

Milk and Yogurt

RECIPES

✈ Shrimp and Corn Bisque _____ 171

✈ Fruit Shakes _____ 172

Yogurt Cheese _____ 173

✈ Soy Milk Smoothie _____ 175

Milk and milk products nutritionally are quite different from the other food groups. A serving from this group provides both carbohydrate and protein. A cup of milk has as much carbohydrate as a slice of bread and as much protein as one ounce of meat.

In addition, few other foods provide such a concentrated source of calcium that is as readily absorbed as do milk, milk products, and calcium-fortified milk substitutes such as soy milk.

Some plants contain calcium, but some also contain substances, such as phytate, oxalate, and fiber, that reduce the amount of calcium absorbed by the body. For example, oxalates are found in spinach, rhubarb, and beet greens. To get the same amount of calcium that you can absorb from 1 cup of milk, you'd need to eat 8 cups of spinach.

The calcium from some vegetables such as broccoli, bok choy, and kale is absorbed as well as or better than calcium from milk and milk products, but these foods have much less calcium per serving. Therefore, without milk and milk-type products, it can be difficult to meet your calcium needs.

The recommended calcium intake is 1,000 to 1,500 milligrams per day, depending on your age and life stage. Getting enough calcium throughout life, and particularly after age 30, helps slow bone loss. Preserving bone mass helps reduce your risk of developing the bone-thinning disease called osteoporosis.

Eight ounces of milk (not calcium-fortified) and 6 ounces of nonfat plain yogurt each provide about 300 milligrams of calcium. Two to three servings of milk, yogurt, or calcium-fortified milk substitutes (1 cup of milk or 6 ounces of yogurt) per day gives you 600 to 900 milligrams of calcium. You will pick up a little more calcium from other calcium-containing foods, such as cheese (found in the meat and meat substitute group) and leafy greens.

You can see it's not easy to get the calcium you need. Because many Americans get too little calcium, more foods are being fortified with calcium.

In a number of regions in the country, dairies are fortifying fat-free milk with calcium to the level of 400 mg or 500 mg per 8 ounces. Some fat-free lactose-reduced milk is also being fortified with calcium.

Calcium-fortified milks are not available country-wide. Check for these products in your area and use them if available. If you don't see them at your supermarket, ask the manager if they can be stocked. Some yogurt and some cheeses are also calcium-fortified. Milk substitutes, such as soy and rice milk, come in calcium-fortified versions but aren't as high in calcium as calcium-fortified milk.

You can also find calcium-fortified juices: orange, grapefruit, and a few others. You can get up to 350 milligrams per 8 ounces, which is 35% of the Daily Value (DV). Some dry cereals are fortified with calcium. Many more calcium-fortified foods will probably become available.

"CALCIUM FORTIFY" MEALS YOURSELF

- When you prepare rice, couscous, or other grains where the moisture soaks in during cooking, substitute milk for water. This fortifies the grain with more calcium.

- Add dry milk to recipes where the taste will blend in: meat loaf or meatballs, soups, casseroles, gravies.

- Add fat-free milk or dry milk to eggs mixed for scrambled eggs, omelettes, or French toast.

- When you make hot cereal, use milk in place of at least half (if not all) the water. Use more milk on the cereal as you eat it.

- Eat more high-fiber cold cereal. It's a way to drink more milk and get a good boost of fiber. Choose a cereal that is calcium-fortified.

- Don't limit cereal and milk to breakfast. It can be a quick and easy lunch, dinner, or snack. Top it with fruit to fit in one more fruit serving.

- Blend up a milk or yogurt shake for a quick and healthy snack. (See recipe, p. 175)

- Create your own yogurt combo. Take plain, fat-free yogurt or frozen yogurt and toss in Grape Nuts or low-fat granola cereal and diced, dried apricots, apples, or pears. A few (just a few) nuts add good crunch.

- Drop a few tablespoons of yogurt on fresh or canned fruit.

- Use plain yogurt as a substitute for sour cream on potatoes. Mix in fresh herbs, garlic, Dijon mustard, cayenne, or curry (or any combination) for some extra kick.

- Make a yogurt dip and enjoy with fresh vegetables or fruit. If you don't like yogurt, blenderize cottage cheese and use that for dips.

- Keep containers of nonfat yogurt in the refrigerator to use as a quick and convenient snack or part of a meal.

- Make custard or pudding for a snack or dessert.

- Enjoy hot cocoa. Make it with fat-free milk.

- Make soup with a combination of milk and water.

BEYOND CALCIUM

Milk and yogurt also have riboflavin, magnesium, phosphorus, and potassium. And milk and yogurt have vitamin B12.

Milk is also a good source of vitamin A and an excellent source of vitamin D. The United States Department of Agriculture, the agency that regulates milk and dairy foods, requires that all milk be fortified with vitamin D and that reduced-fat milk (1% and 2% milk) be fortified with vitamin A. Reduced-fat milk is fortified with vitamin A because vitamin A is in the fat portion of milk, which is removed to produce reduced-fat milks. Reduced-fat milks are required to be fortified with vitamin A to a level found in whole milk, which is 300 IU per 8 ounces. Dairy processors are being encouraged to fortify lower-fat milks to 500 IU of vitamin A per 8 ounces, which is 10% of the Daily Value.

10 EXCELLENT SOURCES OF CALCIUM

Food	Serving	Calcium (mg)
Milk, fat-free, calcium-fortified	1 cup	400–500
Milk, all types of cow's	1 cup	300
Soy milk, calcium-fortified	1 cup	300
Yogurt, all types	3/4 cup/6 oz	250–300
Hard cheeses, all types	1 oz	200–300
Custard, pudding	1/2 cup	150–200
Orange juice, calcium-fortified (35%)	1/2 cup	175
Hot cocoa mix, low-calorie	1 package	100 (range 50–150)
Greens: collard, kale, turnip, spinach	1/2 cup cooked	100 (range 50–150)
Tofu	1/2 cup	130

Many soy milks are fortified with calcium and vitamins A and D to the levels found in cow's milk.

One drawback to milk and yogurt is that they are of animal origin and their full-fat forms contain saturated fat and cholesterol. Luckily, milk and yogurt are both available in fat-free forms.

Soy milks, even the full-fat versions, don't have any cholesterol. You can also buy soy yogurts.

CAN'T HANDLE LACTOSE?

Do you have cramps, bloating, gas, diarrhea, and nausea after eating or drinking cow's milk products? You may be lactose intolerant, meaning you can't digest lactose, the sugar in milk and dairy products. Symptoms begin about 30 minutes to 2 hours after eating or drinking foods containing lactose. The severity of symptoms depends on the amount of lactose consumed and the amount a person can tolerate.

Between 30 and 50 million Americans are lactose intolerant. A large percentage of African Americans, Native Americans, and Asian-Americans are lactose intolerant. The condition is least common among people of northern European descent. People get more lactose intolerant as they age.

Many people who are intolerant to lactose can drink some milk without developing symptoms. Others, however, are affected after eating much smaller amounts of lactose. If you can tolerate some milk and dairy foods, it is nutritionally wise to eat these. Here are a few other helpful hints to get enough calcium.

- Try calcium-fortified soy milk instead of cow's milk. Soy milk has no lactose.
- Buy lactose-reduced or lactose-free milk. You'll find these with the other milks.
- Get lactase drops and treat your milk at home. Or use lactase tablets, which you take before you eat a meal with lactose.
- Buy other lactose-reduced or lactose-free dairy products, such as cottage cheese.

- Choose yogurt or buttermilk. They may be easier to digest because of their active cultures.
- Eat small amounts of regular dairy foods and eat them with a meal. They are often better tolerated this way.
- If you determine you are just not going to get enough calcium on a daily basis, consider taking a calcium supplement.

CALCIUM BEYOND FOOD

If you have a lactose intolerance, or you know you won't include enough dairy or calcium-fortified foods, or you don't like milk, you need to get your calcium from non-food sources.

Don't rely on a multivitamin for your calcium supply. They don't contain that much calcium because fitting enough calcium in would make the pill too large to swallow.

You'll need to take a separate calcium supplement. Look for a calcium-based antacid, such as Tums, or a calcium supplement that contains vitamin D. Take your calcium supplements between meals so you don't decrease the absorption of iron contained in your meals.

Shrimp and Corn Bisque

Serving Size: about 1 1/4 cups, Total Servings: 4

When you want something creamy to start off your meal or be the meal itself, low-fat cream soups are the answer. Using 1% milk will give you a creamy taste. Fat-free milk will produce a soup that's not as rich-tasting, but you can use it if that's what you have on hand.

1/2 lb medium shrimp, peeled and deveined	**1** cup diced, seeded tomato
2 tsp butter	**1/2** cup diced celery
2 Tbsp unbleached flour	**1/4** cup tomato paste
2 cups fat-free, reduced-sodium chicken broth	**1** cup yellow corn
2 cups 1% milk	**2** tsp dry sherry
1 cup chopped onion	**1/4** tsp salt
	1/4 tsp black pepper

1 Coarsely chop the shrimp and set aside.

2 In a 3-quart saucepan, melt the butter over medium heat. Add the flour and cook for 1 minute. Add the broth and milk and bring to a boil. Lower the heat, and add the onion, tomato, celery, and tomato paste. Cook for 3 minutes.

3 Add the corn and reserved shrimp. Cook for 3 minutes until shrimp is cooked through. Add the sherry, salt, and pepper. Serve.

PREPARATION
15 minutes

COOK
10 minutes

Exchanges
2 Carbohydrate
1 Lean Meat

Calories 207
   Calories from Fat 38
Total Fat . . . . 4 g
   Saturated Fat . . . . 2 g
Cholesterol . . . . 83 mg
Sodium . . . . 581 mg
Carbohydrate . . . . 27 g
   Dietary Fiber . . . . 3 g
   Sugars . . . . .11 g
Protein . . . . .16 g

Fruit Shakes

Serving Size: about 1 cup, Total Servings: 2

A nice snack or quick breakfast. The blender does the work, you get the taste!

Basic Mix

- **1** cup fat-free milk
- **1** cup chopped fresh fruit (see fruit options)
- **1** tsp vanilla
- **2** tsp honey
- **3–4** large ice cubes

Fruit Options

- **1** banana, peeled
- **1** cup strawberries, stemmed and washed
- **1** cup cut-up peaches
- **1** cup blueberries

1 Put all ingredients into a blender and blend until smooth.

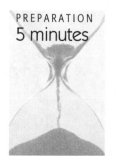

PREPARATION
5 minutes

Exchanges
1 Fruit
1/2 Milk, fat-free

Calories 107
   Calories from Fat 4
Total Fat . . . . 0 g
   Saturated Fat . . . . 0 g
Cholesterol . . . . 2 mg
Sodium . . . . 65 mg
Carbohydrate . . . . 22 g
   Dietary Fiber . . . . 2 g
   Sugars . . . . 18 g
Protein . . . . 5 g

Yogurt Cheese

Serving Size: 2 Tbsp, Total Servings: 4

Have a yen for cheese without the fat? Try yogurt cheese you make yourself. All the whey gets drained from the yogurt producing a creamy yogurt not unlike cream cheese. Add different flavorings from the list below and you can create your own yogurt cheese bar!

1 cup fat-free yogurt

1 Cut a piece of cheesecloth to fit a fine mesh strainer or sieve. Put the strainer in a bowl.

2 Add the yogurt and cover with plastic wrap. Refrigerate overnight until most of the liquid drains out of the yogurt.

3 Use the yogurt cheese on toast, potatoes, and more!

Variations:

After the yogurt has drained, add by hand one of the following:

Herb: 1 Tbsp minced herb of choice (basil, thyme, and dill are great)

Sweet: 2 Tbsp no-sugar jam of choice

Nutty: 2 Tbsp chopped toasted almonds, walnuts

Fruity: 1/4 cup chopped strawberries or raspberries

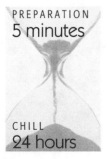

PREPARATION
5 minutes

CHILL
24 hours

Onion: 2 Tbsp finely minced onion and 2 tsp minced parsley

Exchanges
Free food

Calories 16
  Calories from Fat 0
Total Fat . . . . 0 g
  Saturated Fat . . . . 0 g
Cholesterol . . . . 0 mg
Sodium . . . . 20 mg
Carbohydrate . . . . 2 g
  Dietary Fiber . . . . 0 g
  Sugars . . . . 1 g
Protein . . . . 2 g

Exchanges, Yogurt Cheese, Nutty Variation
1/2 Fat

Calories 40
  Calories from Fat 19
Total Fat . . . . 2 g
  Saturated Fat . . . . 0 g
Cholesterol . . . . 0 mg
Sodium . . . . 21 mg
Carbohydrate . . . . 3 g
  Dietary Fiber . . . . 1 g
  Sugars . . . . 1 g
Protein . . . . 2 g

Soy milk, fortified with vitamins A, D, B12, and calcium

Soy milk is a good source of soy protein (7 to 8 grams per cup), thiamine, iron, phosphorus, copper, potassium, and magnesium. It contains very little sodium. Depending on the brand, fortified soy milk can be an excellent source of certain vitamins and calcium. Soy milk has no cholesterol.

How to Buy and Store

Soy milk is available in most grocery stores. You can buy it in aseptic packages that don't need to be refrigerated until the package is opened. These are usually stocked near the evaporated milk or other packaged beverages. Once opened, it stays fresh in the refrigerator for about five days.

You'll also find soy milk in typical milk containers in the refrigerated section with cow's milk. Soy milk is also sold as a powder you can mix with water. Store soy milk powder in the refrigerator or freezer.

Read the label! Make sure you buy a soy milk fortified with calcium and vitamins, especially if you're drinking soy milk as a substitute for cow's milk.

Soy milk is available fat-free or with a higher fat and calorie content. It's also available with flavors. Flavoring adds calories and carbohydrate.

Soy Milk Smoothie

Serving Size: about 1 cup, Total Servings: 4

This recipe calls for a frozen banana. Peel the banana, wrap in wax paper, and freeze. You may opt to use a fresh banana instead, the smoothie will just not be as thick. This is one of the best ways we know of incorporating more soy into your food plan. The berries and banana add the flavor you need to enjoy this as a midday snack or as a breakfast beverage.

3 cups calcium-fortified, plain or vanilla soy milk

1 banana, peeled and frozen

1 cup berries of choice

1 tsp almond or vanilla extract

1 Blend all ingredients until smooth.

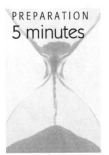

PREPARATION
5 minutes

Exchanges
1/2 Fruit
1/2 Milk, reduced-fat
1/2 Fat

Calories 104
   Calories from Fat 34
Total Fat . . . . 4 g
   Saturated Fat . . . . 0 g
Cholesterol . . . . 0 mg
Sodium . . . . 24 mg
Carbohydrate . . . . .14 g
   Dietary Fiber . . . . 4 g
   Sugars . . . . 8 g
Protein . . . . 6 g

SECTION 7

Milk and Milk Products

	Exchange/ Serving	Calories	Carbohydrate (g)	Protein (g)	Total Fat (g)	Sat. Fat (g)	Cholesterol (mg)
Nonfat or very low-fat							
Buttermilk, low-fat/fat-free	1 cup	99	12	8	2	1.5	9
Evaporated fat-free milk	1/2 cup	100	14	10	0.5	0	5
Milk, dry, fat-free	1/3 cup	82	12	8	0	0	4
Milk, fat-free	1 cup	86	12	8	0.5	0.5	4
Milk, 1%	1 cup	102	12	8	2.5	1.5	10
Yogurt, nonfat, plain	3/4 cup (6 oz)	90	13	10	0	0	4
Yogurt, nonfat, fruit-flavored, nonnutritive sweetener	1 cup	100	17	9	0	0	4
Low-fat							
Milk, 2%	1 cup	121	12	8	4.5	3	18
Sweet Acidophilus milk	1 cup	110	12	8	3.5	2.5	15
Yogurt, low-fat, plain	3/4 cup (6 oz)	112	13	10	3	2	15
Whole							
Whole milk	1 cup	150	11	8	8	5	33
Evaporated milk	1/2 cup	169	13	9	10	6	37
Goat's milk, whole	1 cup	168	11	9	10	6.5	28

Blood Pressure

The evidence continues to grow that control of blood pressure is just as important as control of blood glucose in people with diabetes. Controlling both blood pressure and blood glucose lowers your risk of strokes, and heart, eye, and kidney disease.

The American Diabetes Association recommends that you have your blood pressure checked at every medical visit. Blood pressure for people 18 years of age or older and not pregnant should be under 130 mmHg systolic (top number) and under 80 mmHg diastolic (bottom number).

If your blood pressure is higher than this, try to lose some weight (if you are overweight), reduce your intake of sodium and alcohol, and increase your level of activity. If these strategies don't decrease blood pressure, then your health care provider should start you on a blood pressure medication. Today the preferred blood pressure medication for people with diabetes is an ACE-inhibitor because it not only controls blood pressure, but it also helps protect the kidney from damage.

Sodium and Blood Pressure: What's the Relationship?

Many people think that lowering sodium intake will decrease anyone's high blood pressure. That's not true. People differ in their sensitivity to sodium and its effect on their blood pressure. It's thought that only about 30% of Americans have blood pressure that is sensitive to their sodium intake, that is, if they decrease their sodium intake, their blood pressure will decrease.

If you have high blood pressure, try limiting your sodium intake to see if that change lowers your blood pressure.

The recommendation on sodium intake for healthy people with diabetes is the same as for the general public: between 2,400 and 3,000 mg per day. If you have mild to moderately high blood pressure, lower your sodium intake to 2,400 mg or less per day. If you have high blood pressure and kidney disease from diabetes, lower your sodium intake to 2,000 mg or less per day. To give you a frame of reference, most adult Americans consume between 4,000 and 6,000 mg of sodium a day.

Salt and Sodium: The Same?

You often hear the words salt and sodium used interchangeably. However, they aren't the same thing. Table salt is sodium chloride. It's 40% sodium and 60% chloride. One teaspoon of salt contains 2,300 milligrams of sodium. That's nearly a day's supply of sodium.

It's easy to find the sodium content of packaged foods because the sodium is provided on the food label's Nutrition Facts. Make sure you note the serving size as well as the sodium content because the sodium is listed per one serving.

Cream of Mushroom Soup

Nutrition Facts
Serving Size: 1/2 cup (120 ml)
                condensed soup
Servings per Container: About 2.5

	AMOUNT PER SERVING
Calories	.70
Calories from Fat	25

	% DAILY VALUE
Total Fat 2.5g	2%
Saturated Fat 1g	2%
Cholesterol less than 5mg	1%
Sodium 790mg	33%
Total Carbohydrate 10g	3%
Dietary Fiber <1g	3%
Sugars 2g	0%
Protein 1g	0%

A DASH of News

Sodium does affect blood pressure in some people, but focusing only on sodium gives too narrow a view of how diet affects blood pressure. The DASH Study has done much to broaden the view.

Dietary **A**pproaches to **S**top **H**ypertension was a multi-center study conducted by the National Heart, Lung, and Blood Institute of the National Institutes of Health to test the effects of three different eating plans on blood pressure in 459 people, average age 45. Nearly 60% of the people were minorities and nearly 50% were women.

There were three eating plans: usual American diet, a diet high in fruit and vegetables, and the combination diet that was high in fruits, vegetables, low-fat dairy products, and other reduced-fat foods.

The combination diet significantly lowered blood pressures. Systolic pressure, which at the start was 140–159 mmHg, went down an average of 11 points. Diastolic pressure, which at the start of the study was 90–99 mmHg, went down an average of 5.5 points.

The diet high in fruits and vegetables showed about half the effect of lowering blood pressure compared with the combination diet.

Amazingly, the effect of the diet was evident within one week! Blood pressure was maximally lowered in two weeks and stayed lowered as long as the combination diet was continued.

It's thought that the plan was effective because of the emphasis on vegetables, fruits, and low-fat dairy products high in calcium.

The men and women in the study achieved similar blood pressure reductions. People who had high blood pressure at the beginning of the study had a greater lowering of their blood pressure than people with normal blood pressure.

What to Eat to Do the DASH

- 4–5 servings of vegetables daily (a serving is 1/2 cup cooked vegetables, 1 cup raw leafy vegetables, or 6 oz vegetable juice)

- 4–5 servings of fruit daily (a serving is 1 medium fruit, 1/4 cup dried fruit, 1/2 cup fresh, frozen, or canned fruit, or 6 oz juice)

- 7–8 daily servings of grains (a serving is one slice of bread, 1/2 cup cooked rice or pasta, or 1/2 cup dry cereal)

- 2–3 daily servings of dairy foods, nonfat or low-fat

(a serving is 1 cup milk or yogurt, 1.5 oz cheese)

- 2 or fewer daily servings (3 oz) of fish, poultry, or lean meat

- 4–5 weekly servings of nuts, seeds, and beans (1/3 cup nuts, 2 Tbsp seeds, 1/2 cup cooked beans)

These servings apply to people who require 2,000 calories per day. The number of servings may increase or decrease depending on your caloric needs, which vary according to age, gender, size, and how active you are. The diet should be changed by lowering the number of servings of grains but not fruits and vegetables.

For further information on the DASH diet, go to the website:

http://DASH.bwh.harvard.edu

FOODS TO LIMIT
The salt shaker
Processed and prepared foods
Snack foods
Fast foods and restaurant meals
Bacon and sausage
Canned soups
Cold cuts: ham, bologna, salami, corned beef
Condiments: olives, pickles, sauerkraut
Soy and teriyaki sauce, low-fat
   salad dressings

Meat and Meat Substitutes

RECIPES

SOY

✈ Roasted Soy Nuts _____ 195

✈ Teriyaki Tofu Kabobs _____ 196

SEAFOOD, FISH

✈ Chinese Ginger Salmon _____ 199

✈ Seared Salmon with Asparagus
and Green Onion _____ 200

✈ Seared Sesame Tuna
with Orange Glaze _____ 201

✈ Teriyaki Glazed Tuna _____ 202

✈ Middle Eastern Tuna Salad _____ 203

✈ 4 Ways with Tuna or Salmon _____ 204

Crunchy Shrimp
and Broccoli Stir-Fry _____ 206

Cioppino _____ 207

Seafood Kabobs Hawaiian _____ 208

Stir-Fry Fish _____ 209

New Orleans Shrimp Creole _____ 210

Shrimp Scampi _____ 211

Crispy Fish Filets _____ 212

Low-Fat Sauces for Fish:
Tartar Sauce, Cold Cucumber Sauce _____ 213

CHICKEN, TURKEY

Wild Rice Sun-dried Cherry
Stuffed Chicken_____ 216

Chicken with Tri-colored Peppers _____ 218

Grilled Chicken Breasts
with Fruit Salsa _____ 219

Chicken Salad in 64+ Ways _____ 220

Oriental Turkey Salad _____ 222

RED MEAT

Marinated Steak Kabobs _____ 225

Chinese Stir-Fried Beef with Ginger_____ 226

Spiced Lamb Stew_____ 227

This section of the pyramid houses foods with a hefty dose of protein. It includes meat, seafood, cheese, eggs, and soy products.

One exchange, which for most of the foods is a 1-oz serving, has 7 grams of protein and 0 grams of carbohydrate. There's no carbohydrate, so you might expect that it won't raise your blood glucose. But when fat is also in the serving, it can just slow down the rise and surprise you with high blood glucose hours after the meal.

The foods are grouped according to how much fat they contain.

- Very lean
- Lean
- Medium-fat
- High-fat

Very lean

0–1 grams fat, 35 calories per exchange

Examples: Skinless chicken breast, tuna canned in water, low-fat cottage cheese, egg whites. In addition, a serving of dried peas or beans counts as 1 very lean meat exchange and 1 starch.

Lean

3 grams fat, 55 calories

Examples: Sirloin steak trimmed of fat, salmon, catfish

Medium-fat

5 grams fat, 75 calories

Examples: Ground beef, pork chop, fried fish, mozzarella cheese, whole egg, tofu. (Unlike the other members of this group, tofu has no cholesterol.)

High-fat

8 grams fat, 100 calories

Examples: Country pork ribs and regular cheese

For healthy eating, keep three things in mind when choosing foods from the protein section:

- **Eat smaller portions and fewer servings.** Strive for two to three 3-oz cooked servings each day. That's likely less than you've been eating.

- **Choose more of your protein foods from the very lean and lean groups.** Most of the protein foods are of animal origin and contain various amounts of saturated fat and cholesterol. Choosing from the very lean or lean sections means less saturated fat, less total fat, and fewer calories.

- **Make more of your protein choices tofu or certain types of fish** (the Nutrition Superstars for this chapter).

LIGHTEN UP ON PROTEIN

Food choices today channel you toward protein, and usually animal sources of protein. Think about the daily question: "What's for dinner? Beef, chicken, or fish?" At a fast food spot, it's hamburger or grilled chicken. Even in the supermarket, frozen entrees focus on protein: glazed chicken with rice and carrots, chopped beef steak with potatoes and green beans.

But you just don't need as much protein as the typical American gets. And you certainly don't need the artery-clogging saturated fat that goes along with many of the animal-based protein foods.

Break out of the American mold! Strive for the adult RDA for protein of 0.4 grams per pound of body weight per day. That's not much—about 60 to 65 grams of protein for the average man and about 50 to 55 grams of protein for the average woman. That's two to three 3-oz cooked servings of meat or meat substitutes per day. And everyone can benefit from choosing more vegetable sources of protein instead of animal.

Here's a sample menu for 0.4 grams of protein per pound (60–65 grams) for a man eating 1,800–2,000 calories a day.

BREAKFAST

Food	Amount	Calories	Protein (g)
Cereal	1 1/2 cups	160	6
Milk, fat-free	3/4 cup	65	6
Banana	1 small	60	0
Blueberries	3/4 cup	60	0
Yogurt, plain	1/4 cup	30	2

LUNCH

Food	Amount	Calories	Protein (g)
Vegetable soup	1 cup	80	3
Bread	2 slices	160	6
Smoked turkey	1 oz	35	7
Swiss cheese, part skim	1 oz	75	3
Avocado, sliced	1/8	45	0
Lettuce, tomato for sandwich	1 cup	12	2
Mayonnaise, regular	2 tsp	90	0
Cantaloupe	1 cup cubed	60	0

DINNER

Food	Amount	Calories	Protein (g)
Tofu	1/2 cup	75	7
Stir-fry vegetables	1 1/2 cups	75	6
Canola oil	3 tsp	135	0
Rice	1 cup	240	9
Raspberries and blueberries	1 cup	60	0

SNACK

Food	Amount	Calories	Protein (g)
Crackers	1 serving	80	3
Hummus	1/3 cup	125	3
Baby carrots	10	25	2
Salad dressing	2 Tbsp	90	0

Here's a sample menu for 0.4 grams of protein per pound (50–55 grams) for a woman eating 1,400–1,600 calories.

BREAKFAST

Food	Amount	Calories	Protein (g)
Cereal	3/4 cup	80	3
Milk	1/2 cup	43	4
Banana	1 small	60	0
Blueberries	3/4 cup	60	0
Yogurt, plain	1/4 cup	30	2

LUNCH

Food	Amount	Calories	Protein (g)
Vegetable soup	1 cup	80	3
Bread	2 slices	160	6
Smoked turkey	1 oz	35	7
Swiss cheese, part skim	1 oz	75	3
Avocado, sliced	1/8	45	0
Lettuce, tomato for sandwich	1 cup	12	2
Cantaloupe	1 cup, cubed	60	0

DINNER

Food	Amount	Calories	Protein (g)
Tofu	1/2 cup	75	7
Stir-fry vegetables	1 1/2 cups	75	6
Canola oil	2 tsp	90	0
Rice	2/3 cup	160	6
Raspberries and blueberries	1 cup	60	0

SNACK

Food	Amount	Calories	Protein (g)
Crackers	1 serving	80	3
Hummus	1/3 cup	125	3
Baby carrots	10	25	2
Salad dressing	1 Tbsp	45	0

EASY TIPS FOR CUTTING BACK ON MEAT

- If you're used to eating a lot of meat, 3 ounces will seem like just a few bites. Downsize step-by-step. If you usually buy a 13-ounce rib eye (10 ounces cooked), now choose a leaner cut, such as sirloin or flank steak, and buy a 10-ounce steak (7 to 8 ounces cooked). If you usually eat 5 to 6 ounces of turkey in a sandwich, step down to 4 to 5 ounces, then the next month go down to 3 to 4 ounces.

- Make protein s-t-r-e-t-c-h. Look to the dishes from cultures that have long practiced making a small amount of protein feed many mouths: Chinese stir-fry, Mexican burritos, or Japanese sukiyaki.

- Incorporate small servings of protein such as ground beef or turkey sausage in a tomato sauce and serve it over pasta. This accomplishes several nutrition goals: less meat and fat, more starches and vegetables. From time to time take these recipes one step further and eliminate meat all together.

- In restaurants, split sandwiches or share a tuna- or chicken-salad plate. Ask for extra pieces of bread or roll.

- Make your own sandwiches with less protein. Load them with raw vegetables— lettuce, tomato, sliced cucumbers, peppers.

- Take up more room on your plate with filling grains, starches, and vegetables. Leave room for meat only as a side dish.

- Buy smaller quantities so you eat smaller portions. Think about the amount you need at the meat counter so you don't prepare more than you need.

- In fast-food restaurants order single, regular, or junior-size sandwiches. Stay away from the doubles and triples.

- Start your day without a serving of meat. Eat a bowl of cereal, a bagel, or an English muffin for breakfast.

- Gather recipes that de-emphasize meat and emphasize grains and vegetables. Prepare a new one each week or two.

CHOOSE LEAN

Meat and Poultry

There are higher-fat and leaner cuts of all the red meats. The white meat of poultry is lower in fat than the dark meat.

First, choose leaner cuts. Next, trim fat from red meat and remove the skin from poultry. Then cook in ways that get rid of more fat: grilling, broiling, or baking on a rack. And finally, don't add fat back by, for example, breading and deep frying.

Fish

Fish is a safe bet, because it falls into either the very lean or lean groups, unless you fry it. And even when you choose a "fatty" fish such as tuna or salmon, you're getting omega-3 fats, which are good for you. As with meat, use low-fat cooking techniques.

LOW-FAT COOKING TECHNIQUES, SAUCES, AND SEASONING

- Grill with different flavored chips: mesquite, hickory, or applewood.

- Barbecue with barbecue sauce (make a batch of your own or use a commercial one).

- Poach in broth, wine, or sherry, plus garlic or herbs.

- Marinate meat, chicken, or fish for several hours in fat-free ingredients: sherry, mustard, and garlic; soy or teriyaki sauce; ginger and garlic; any variety vinegar.

- Marinate meat, chicken, or fish for several hours in a reduced- or fat-free salad dressing.

- Make low-fat gravy: Take the drippings and get rid of the fat. Put in pan, heat, and add a bit of flour or cornstarch to thicken. Puree any celery, onion, or carrots that were in the roasting pan and add to defatted gravy mixture to thicken.

- For fajitas, burritos, or soft tacos, use salsa or pico de gallo as a topping instead of cheese or sour cream. Try this when you eat these foods in restaurants, too.

- Mix plain low-fat or fat-free yogurt with mustard and dill to top fish before and during cooking.

CHEESE

Cheese is in the meat group because, nutritionally speaking, it more closely resembles meat than it does milk and yogurt. It's a complete protein and contains vitamin A and riboflavin. Cheese differs from meats in that it contains a small amount of carbohydrate, calcium, and sodium. Overall cheese, in small portions, is a healthy food choice.

Today many more cheeses are available in reduced-fat, part-skim, low-fat, and fat-free forms, so you can enjoy cheese while eliminating some fat, saturated fat, and cholesterol. Plus, cheese is not a food you eat in large portions. An ounce here and there is more common, and that's the way it should be.

Enjoy cheese sparingly. Spread it by crumbling or shredding it on salads, casseroles, or pasta. Use cheeses with sharp tastes so you can use less cheese.

THE NUTRITION NUMBERS FOR CHEESE

Cheese/Type	Amount	Calories	Fat (g)	Sat. Fat (g)	Chol. (mg)
American					
Regular	1 oz	106	9	6	27
Reduced-fat	1 oz	68	4	3	14
Low-fat	1 oz	51	2	1	10
Nonfat	1 oz	37	0	0	7
Cheddar					
Regular	1 oz	114	9	6	30
Reduced-fat	1 oz	81	5	4	15
Low-fat	1 oz	49	2	1	6
Nonfat	1 oz	41	0	0	0
Feta					
Regular	1 oz	75	6	4	25
Reduced-fat	1 oz	61	4	3	10
Mozzarella					
Regular	1 oz	90	7	4	25
Part-skim	1 oz	80	5	3	15
Fat-free	1 oz	41	0	0	5

(continued)

THE NUTRITION NUMBERS FOR CHEESE (CONTINUED)

Cheese/Type	Amount	Calories	Fat (g)	Sat. Fat (g)	Chol. (mg)
Swiss					
Regular	1 oz	107	8	5	26
Reduced-fat	1 oz	91	6	4	20
Low-fat	1 oz	51	2	1	10
Nonfat	1 oz	41	0	0	0
Parmesan					
Regular	2 Tbsp	57	4	3	10
Nonfat	2 Tbsp	31	0	0	3
Cottage cheese					
2% fat	1/4 cup	51	1	1	5
1% fat	1/4 cup	41	0.5	0	3
Fat-free	1/4 cup	40	0	0	3
Ricotta cheese					
Regular	1/4 cup	107	8	5	31
Part-skim	1/4 cup	85	5	3	19

PORTION CONTROL WITH PROTEIN FOODS

It's easy to go overboard on portions of sliced meat and cheese, because one more ounce doesn't seem like that much more food. However in calories, it's another 35 to 100 calories depending on the fat content of the item.

Try this: When you buy a package of cheese, cold cuts, or anything you buy by the ounce, glance at the ounces on the label. Then visualize what 1 or 2 ounces looks like.

Before you buy cheese or cold cuts sliced to order, think about how many meals you'll be making. Let that number be your guide to the number of ounces you buy. If you make a smoked turkey and Swiss cheese sandwich for lunch, with 2 ounces of turkey and 1 ounce of cheese, how many sandwiches do you need to make until the next time you shop? Buy the amount you need, not just any amount. A side effect of this trick is that you'll waste less food.

Q Does eating a diet high in protein or taking amino acid supplements help build muscles?

A No. This is a widely held and propagated belief in the muscle and fitness community, but it's simply not true. Protein is critical for muscle and bone growth, but eating extra protein doesn't increase muscle growth. Muscles only grow as a result of exercise and an adequate number of calories and nutrition to support the growth.

Q Since I have diabetes, should I follow a low-carbohydrate, high-protein diet?

A No. These are not healthy diets in the short- or long-term.

Some books promote eating very low levels of carbohydrate, even encouraging people not to eat fruit or many servings of starches. Others allow more carbohydrate, but still a lower-than-desirable intake.

Will they help you lower your blood glucose? Yes, temporarily. Are they regimens that most people can follow over the course of months and years? No.

Are they healthy diets? No! They tend to be light in fiber and calcium, and loaded down with protein and fat, particularly saturated fat. More saturated fat is one thing that people with diabetes definitely don't need.

The dietary regimens promoted in these books are not consistent with the nutrition recommendations from American Diabetes Association. In addition, these "fad diets" don't work in the long run. Anyone can follow a regimen for a couple of weeks or months. That's not the issue. What's most important is that you make small gradual changes to improve the healthiness of your food choices and control your blood glucose over the course of time.

Quick fixes don't work. If they did, you wouldn't be hearing about new bestsellers every few years.

Soy Foods

Soy milk, tofu, vegetarian burgers, and more. Soy-based foods are growing in popularity and a greater variety of products are popping up, not just in health food stores but in supermarkets as well.

One reason is mounting research that touts the health benefits of soy. Soybeans contain a variety of phytochemicals, and they are the only food with a significant amount of isoflavones.

Isoflavones are chemically similar in structure to estrogen and, in fact, are weak estrogens. The two primary isoflavones in soybeans are daidzein and genistein. Soy-based foods typically contain more genistein than daidzein. Soy-based foods differ somewhat in their concentration of isoflavones, but all of the traditional soy foods, such as tofu, soy milk, tempeh, and miso, are good sources of isoflavones, providing about 30 to 40 milligrams per serving.

Research on the benefits of isoflavones from soy-based foods has shown that they may lower total cholesterol and LDL ("bad") cholesterol, decrease the breakdown of bones that leads to osteoporosis, and diminish the risk of some cancers including breast and prostate cancer.

The only research that is thus far considered absolute is the benefit of isoflavones in heart disease. Because of this research, late in 1999 the FDA approved the first food labeling health claim about soy. The claim can read: "Soy protein, as part of a diet low in saturated fat and cholesterol, may reduce the risk for coronary heart disease." Foods that carry the claim must provide 6.25 grams of soy per serving and also meet the requirements for low fat, low saturated fat, and low cholesterol content except the foods made with the whole soybean. The amount of soy per serving is based on research that shows that to realize soy's heart benefits you must eat 25 grams of soy protein per day.

Soy protein is available from soy milk, soybeans, soy flour, sweet green soybeans (edamama), tofu, and soy nuts.

To eat 25 grams of soy a day you definitely have to work at it. You can't just have a cup of soy milk or a serving of tofu a day to get the benefits to your blood fats. You need to regularly include several servings each day of soy-based foods such as soy flour to make pancakes or waffles, soy milk, soy-based yogurt, soy-based cereals, soy cheese and cream cheese, soy nuts, tofu and tempeh, and commercially available soy-based products.

Soy sauce and soy oil don't contain isoflavones. Also, soy protein concentrates, which are made with an alcohol extraction process, have low concentrations of isoflavones and may not have the same protective effects as soy-based foods.

Isoflavone supplements, in capsule form, are widely available and growing in popularity. However numerous studies have failed to document health benefits associated with the use of soy supplement. It appears that both soy protein and its isoflavones are necessary for the full health benefits.

Tofu

Tofu is made by curdling hot soy milk. It's also known as soybean curd. Tofu is low in saturated fat and has no cholesterol. Light tofu is available in most supermarkets and is lower in fat.

Tofu can be a good source of calcium. One of the curdling agents that can be used to make tofu is calcium salt. Some tofu manufacturers fortify tofu with calcium. Check the label to see how much calcium is present.

There are different types of tofu. They vary by firmness, texture, and amount of protein.

- Extra-firm tofu contains less water and maintains its shape very well, making it ideal for slicing, cubing, stir-frying, broiling, and grilling. Extra-firm tofu contains more protein and fat than the other forms. It can be frozen and thawed, which gives it a more meat-like texture, then added to casseroles, lasagna, or spaghetti sauce in place of red meat.

- Firm tofu is not as dense, though it also holds its shape for slicing, cubing, and stir-frying. Firm tofu works well in dips, and as a cheese substitute, particularly for cottage cheese, ricotta, or cream cheese.

- Soft tofu is much less dense. It's ideal for blending into salad dressings and sauces. It can be used to reduce or replace sour cream or yogurt. Soft tofu is lower in both protein and fat.

- Silken tofu has a much finer consistency than other forms of tofu. Silken tofu is available in extra firm, firm, and soft.

How to Store

Most brands of tofu are found in the produce section, where they can be kept cool. This type of tofu needs to be refrigerated at home as well. Aseptically packaged tofu is also available; it needs no refrigeration until it is opened. Once opened, use quickly or store in fresh changes of water for 3 days.

Tempeh

Tempeh is a cultured soybean cake. It has a tender, chewy consistency that makes it versatile as a meat substitute. Tempeh can be grilled, sauteed, steamed, baked, grated, or microwaved. It holds its shape well.

Tempeh is becoming more common in mainstream grocery stores, usually in the frozen food section. Frozen, packaged tempeh stays fresh for at least a year. Once thawed and opened, it stays fresh in the refrigerator for about one month.

Tempeh is a good source of high-quality protein because it's soy-based. It's low in saturated fats and has no cholesterol. It's also an excellent source of dietary fiber; one 3-oz serving of tempeh contains over 6 grams of dietary fiber. Tempeh is also a good source of calcium, some B vitamins, and iron.

Tips for Tasty Tofu and Tempeh

- Add chunks of firm tofu or tempeh to soups, stews, and casseroles.

- Stir-fry with tofu or tempeh. Use it instead of or to reduce the amount of red meat, poultry, or fish.

- Mix crumbled tofu or tempeh into a meat loaf to decrease the red meat and lighten up the meat loaf. Do the same with hamburgers.

- Mash tofu with cottage cheese or ricotta cheese and seasoning to make a sandwich spread.

- Marinate slices of tofu in barbecue sauce, teriyaki, or soy sauce and grill them.

- Blend soft or silken tofu with seasonings or a package of dry soup mix for a dip.

- Stir silken tofu into reduced-fat sour cream for a low-fat baked potato topper.

- Substitute pureéd silken tofu when dip or salad dressing recipes call for mayonnaise, sour cream, cream cheese, or ricotta cheese.

- Prepare scrambled tofu (use firm) instead of scrambled eggs, or use half tofu and half eggs.

Roasted Soy Nuts

Serving Size: 2 Tbsp, Total Servings: 8

This on-the-go snack is a clever way to get more soy into your food plan. Making your own soy nuts is very easy and less expensive than store-bought soy nuts. You can also regulate the amount of salt used. Try adding any dried herbs and spices such as basil or curry to give the nuts a different taste. You can find dried soybeans in natural food stores.

1 cup dried soybeans	Vegetable-oil cooking spray
1 quart cold water	Salt to taste

1 Rinse beans thoroughly in several changes of cold water. Sort and discard any stone or debris. Put beans in a bowl and cover with 1 quart of cold water. Soak 3–4 hours at room temperature or overnight in the refrigerator. Drain and pat dry.

2 Preheat oven to 350°F. Spray a baking sheet with vegetable oil. Place beans in a single layer on a baking sheet. Bake 35–45 minutes, stirring every 15 minutes, until well browned. Add salt if desired.

3 Transfer to a bowl to cool. Store in a covered container in the refrigerator. Eat as a snack or sprinkle on soups, casseroles, salads.

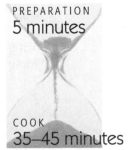

PREPARATION
5 minutes

COOK
35–45 minutes

Exchanges
1/2 Starch
1 Very Lean Meat
1 Fat

Calories 112
   Calories from Fat 52
Total Fat . . . . 6 g
   Saturated Fat . . . . 1 g
Cholesterol . . . . 0 mg
Sodium . . . . 1 mg
Carbohydrate . . . . 6 g
   Dietary Fiber . . . . 4 g
   Sugars . . . . 2 g
Protein . . . . .11 g

Teriyaki Tofu Kabobs

Serving Size: 2 skewers, Total Servings: 4

Be sure to use only extra-firm tofu for this recipe, which will hold up against the heat of the grill. The tofu will take on a slight meat-like consistency making this a nice, healthful change from beef kabobs. Remember that tofu is a relatively bland food; the flavor of added ingredients will be pronounced.

8 bamboo skewers

3/4 lb extra firm tofu, drained and cut into 32 cubes

1 red pepper, cut into 16 squares

1 cup canned pineapple chunks, reserve 1/2 cup juice

1 Tbsp lite soy sauce

1 clove garlic, minced

2 tsp minced ginger

1 Soak skewers in water for 30 minutes to keep them from burning as you cook the skewers.

2 Meanwhile, put the tofu, red pepper, and pineapple chunks in a plastic bag or container with a lid. Add reserved pineapple juice, soy sauce, garlic, and ginger. Marinate for at least 30 minutes.

3 Drain, reserving marinade to baste. Thread the tofu, red pepper, and pineapple on the skewers.

4 Prepare an outdoor grill or oven broiler with the rack set 6 inches from the heat source. Grill or broil the kabobs about 5 minutes per side, basting with the marinade. Serve with brown rice.

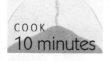

PREPARATION
20 minutes, and
30 minutes marinating time

COOK
10 minutes

Exchanges
1 Carbohydrate
1 Very Lean Meat

Calories 107
  Calories from Fat 15
Total Fat . . . . .2 g
  Saturated Fat . . . . .0 g
Cholesterol . . . . .0 mg
Sodium . . . . .147 mg
Carbohydrate . . . . .17 g
  Dietary Fiber . . . . .2 g
  Sugars . . . . .14 g
Protein . . . . .7 g

Seafood

Both lean and fatty fish are good for you. Lean fish such as sole and flounder are lower in total fat compared with tuna or salmon. On the other hand, salmon and tuna have more of the heart-healthy omega-3 fatty acids. Consider eating a variety of both lean and fatty fish for nutrition as well as for a variety in taste.

There are so many varieties to choose from, shopping for fish with confidence will take some practice.

How to Buy

First, plan seafood into your meal plan. Unlike poultry and meat, fish really tastes best when not frozen, but rather purchased and consumed the same or the next day. If you have to freeze fish, follow the guidelines below.

Always buy fish from a reputable vendor, who will have the equipment to keep fish at its proper temperature. Although the price is right, buying from a roadside stand with no visible signs of proper temperature control could spell trouble.

Fresh Fish: When you buy whole fish, look for bright, clear eyes; red gills; and bright, tight scales or shiny skin. Stale fish have cloudy, sunken eyes. With age, gill color fades to light pink.

The flesh should be firm and springy. Fresh filets or steaks should have flesh that appears to be freshly cut, without a dried or brown look, that is firm in texture. Ask to see your fish out of the case. There should be no "fishy" or ammonia smell.

Ask for your fish to be placed in a bag of ice for the trip home, no matter how close you live to the store. This will keep the fish fresh for the ride home.

Frozen Filets: Wrapping should be of moisture- and vapor-proof material. There should be little or no odor. Look for solidly frozen fish with clear color, free of ice crystals. Discoloration, a brownish tinge, or a covering of ice crystals all indicate that the fish may have been thawed and refrozen.

How to Store

Fresh: Remove fish from original wrapper and rewrap in plastic wrap or a plastic bag. Place package of fish in a dish, cover with ice. Store fish in refrigerator and use within 24 hours. To freeze: Dip the fish in lemon juice to help preserve its original taste and texture. Then wrap it snugly in plastic wrap, followed by a layer of aluminum foil.

Frozen: Keep in the original wrapper; use immediately after thawing. Never thaw and refreeze fish, since this will cause moisture loss, and texture and flavor changes.

How to Thaw

The best way to thaw frozen fish is to leave it in its wrappings and thaw it in the refrigerator or in cold water. Thawing at room temperature may make it soggy. Drain well and blot dry with paper towels.

Seafood high in omega-3 fats

Salmon

A 3-oz serving provides 2 grams of omega-3 fats. Also an excellent source of phosphorus, selenium, riboflavin, niacin, B6, B12. A good source of pantothenic acid, copper, and thiamin.

Tuna, white, canned in water

A 3-oz serving provides 1 gram omega-3 fat. Excellent source of vitamin D and selenium. Good source of vitamin B12 and phosphorus.

Chinese Ginger Salmon

Serving Size: one filet, about 4 ounces, Total Servings: 4

This very quick marinade further deepens the rich flavor of salmon. Soy, ginger, and garlic are enhanced with the techniques of broiling or grilling. Use this marinade for any other fatty fish, such as tuna or swordfish.

4 (4-oz) salmon filets

Marinade

3 Tbsp lite soy sauce

1 tsp sesame oil

2 tsp honey

1 Tbsp dry sherry

1 cup fat-free, reduced-sodium chicken broth

2 tsp minced ginger

1 tsp minced garlic

1 In a large bowl or plastic zippered plastic bag, combine all marinade ingredients.

2 Add the salmon filets and let marinate for 30 minutes or up to 2 hours in the refrigerator.

3 Preheat an oven broiler or outdoor grill with the rack 6 inches from the heat source. Broil or grill the salmon 6 inches from the heat source, for about 8–10 minutes until the fish just turns opaque.

PREPARATION
10 minutes, and
30 minutes to 2 hours marinating time

COOK
10 minutes

Exchanges
3 Lean Meat
1/2 Fat

Calories 201
Calories from Fat 91
Total Fat . . . . .10 g
Saturated Fat . . . . .3 g
Cholesterol . . . . .78 mg
Sodium . . . . 250 mg
Carbohydrate . . . . .1 g
Dietary Fiber . . . . .0 g
Sugars . . . . .1 g
Protein . . . . 24 g

Seared Salmon with Asparagus and Green Onion

Serving Size: about 4 ounces, Total Servings: 4

Searing salmon is a wonderful way to get a good crisp. Just sear the salmon until it is golden on each side, but don't overcook it. This is a beautiful presentation and the asparagus, spring onion, and tomatoes are light enough in taste to carry the earthy taste of the salmon.

1 lb salmon, cut into 4 pieces	**6** green onions, sliced into 2-inch lengths
1/4 tsp salt	**1/2** cup chopped tomato
1/4 tsp pepper	**1** Tbsp fresh lemon juice
3 tsp olive oil, divided	**1** tsp minced sage
1 1/2 cups sliced asparagus, cut into 2-inch pieces, tough ends removed	

1 Season the salmon pieces with the salt and pepper. In a nonstick skillet over medium-high heat, heat 2 tsp of the olive oil. Add the salmon filets and sauté on both sides for a total of 6-8 minutes. Remove the salmon from the skillet, set aside, and keep warm.

2 In a pot of boiling water, add the asparagus and boil for 1 minute. Add the green onion and boil 1 more minute. Drain. Splash with cold water. In a bowl, mix together the asparagus, green onion, and chopped tomato.

3 Combine the remaining 1 tsp of the olive oil, the lemon juice, and sage. In the skillet in which you cooked the salmon, add the asparagus, onion, tomato, and the oil and lemon juice mixture. Heat 1 minute.

4 To serve: Put the salmon on a plate. Top with the vegetables. Pour any pan juices on top.

PREPARATION
20 minutes

COOK
10 minutes

Exchanges
4 Lean Meat
1 Vegetable

Calories 246
 Calories from Fat 118
Total Fat . . . . 13 g
 Saturated Fat . . . . 4 g
Cholesterol . . . . 78 mg
Sodium . . . . 218 mg
Carbohydrate . . . . 6 g
 Dietary Fiber . . . . 2 g
 Sugars . . . . 2 g
Protein . . . . 26 g

Seared Sesame Tuna with Orange Glaze

Serving Size: about 4 ounces, Total Servings: 4

Coating fish with sesame seeds provides crunch and nutrition. Sesame seeds are an excellent source of calcium. For a real taste treat, buy black sesame seeds.

2 Tbsp unbleached flour

Salt and pepper to taste

2 Tbsp sesame seeds

4 (4-oz) portions of fresh tuna steak, 1/2-inch thick

1 Tbsp canola oil

Garnish:

2 Tbsp minced green onions

Glaze

1 tsp sesame oil

2 Tbsp lite soy sauce

1/3 cup fresh orange juice

2 tsp fresh lemon juice

2 Tbsp water

Pinch chili powder

2 tsp cornstarch

1 On a large plate, combine the flour, salt, pepper, and sesame seeds. Dredge each tuna steak in the flour-sesame mixture.

2 In a large skillet over medium-high heat, heat the oil. When the oil is hot, add the tuna steaks and sauté on both sides for a total of 10 minutes (less if you want the tuna a bit more pink in the center). Remove the tuna from the skillet and keep warm.

3 Wipe the skillet clean and add the glaze ingredients. Bring to a boil over high heat until the mixture thickens. Serve the glaze with the cooked tuna. Garnish with minced green onions.

PREPARATION
20 minutes

COOK
15 minutes

Exchanges
1/2 Carbohydrate
4 Lean Meat

Calories 257
  Calories from Fat 111
Total Fat . . . . .12 g
  Saturated Fat . . . . .1 g
Cholesterol . . . . 42 mg
Sodium . . . . 347 mg
Carbohydrate . . . . .9 g
  Dietary Fiber . . . . 1 g
  Sugars . . . . 3 g
Protein . . . . 27 g

Teriyaki Glazed Tuna

Serving Size: about 4 oz, Total Servings: 4

Use this marinade on any other type of seafood, or on poultry, pork, or beef. We prefer our tuna on the rare side, but feel free to cook it a bit longer. You may also pan sear the tuna instead of grilling it. Just put the tuna in a nonstick skillet with a bit of canola oil and cook on both sides for a total of 7–8 minutes.

4 (4-oz) portions tuna steak, 1-inch thick

Marinade

1/4	cup lite soy sauce	**1**	tsp minced ginger
2	Tbsp dry sherry	**2**	cloves garlic, minced
2	tsp sesame oil	**1/4**	tsp crushed red pepper flakes (optional)
2	Tbsp orange juice	**1**	Tbsp brown sugar

1 In a medium bowl or in a zippered plastic bag, combine all marinade ingredients.

2 Add the tuna steaks and turn to coat with marinade. Cover and put in the refrigerator. Marinate the tuna for 2 hours.

3 Remove the tuna from the marinade. Discard marinade. Preheat an oven broiler or grill. Place the tuna steaks on a broiler pan or prepare a grill rack by spraying it with nonstick spray.

4 Broil or grill the tuna 4–6 inches from the heat source, turning once for a total cooking time of 7–8 minutes. (Cook a bit longer if you want well-done tuna.)

PREPARATION
10 minutes, and
2 hours marinating time

COOK
7–8 minutes

Exchanges

4 Very Lean Meat
1/2 Fat

Calories 168
Calories from Fat 54
Total Fat . . . . 6 g
Saturated Fat . . . . 0 g
Cholesterol . . . . 42 mg
Sodium . . . . .194 mg
Carbohydrate . . . . 1 g
Dietary Fiber . . . . 0 g
Sugars . . . . 1 g
Protein . . . . 26 g

Middle Eastern Tuna Salad

Serving Size: about 3 1/2 ounces tuna, Total Servings: 4

This salad will have you thinking about tuna salad in a whole new way. We've boosted the fiber and protein content of traditional tuna by adding chickpeas. We like tuna dressed with oil and lemon rather than slathered with mayonnaise. Stuff this salad into a large, hollowed-out tomato and serve with toasted whole-grain pita bread.

2 (7-oz) cans water-packed tuna, drained

1 large cucumber, peeled and diced

1 small red onion, diced

3 medium tomatoes, seeded and diced

1/2 cup cooked canned chickpeas

1 Tbsp olive oil

2 Tbsp fresh lemon juice

1/2 tsp ground cumin

1/4 tsp ground red pepper

2 tsp toasted sesame seeds

1 In a large salad bowl, combine all ingredients. Cover and chill for 1/2 hour.

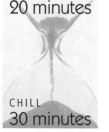

PREPARATION
20 minutes

CHILL
30 minutes

Exchanges

1/2 Starch	3 Very Lean Meat
2 Vegetable	1/2 Fat

Calories 213
   Calories from Fat 48
Total Fat . . . . 5 g
   Saturated Fat . . . . 1 g
Cholesterol . . . . 25 mg
Sodium . . . . 344 mg
Carbohydrate . . . . 15 g
   Dietary Fiber . . . . 4 g
   Sugars . . . . 7 g
Protein . . . . 26 g

4 Ways with Tuna or Salmon
Serving Size: 3 ounces canned tuna or salmon, Total Servings: 4

Here are different ways to prepare tuna or salmon salad apart from the usual fare. Have fun mixing your own combinations. Use a medium salad bowl for the salad, and a small bowl or measuring cup to whisk the dressings. For each variation: Whisk the dressing ingredients. Toss the vegetables with 12 ounces tuna or salmon. Add dressing and toss well. Top with garnish.

Nutrient information was calculated using half tuna and half salmon.

All-American

Dressing

- **1/2** cup low-fat mayonnaise
- **1/4** cup plain nonfat yogurt
- **2** Tbsp lite (reduced-fat) sour cream
- **2** tsp Dijon mustard
  Salt and pepper to taste

Vegetables

- **1/2** cup finely minced onion
- **1/2** cup finely minced celery
- **1/4** cup finely minced red pepper

Exchanges, All American
3 Very Lean Meat
2 Vegetable   1/2 Fat

Calories 189	
Calories from Fat 51	
Total Fat . . . . 6 g	
Saturated Fat . . . . 0 g	
Cholesterol . . . . 39 mg	
Sodium . . . . 751 mg	
Total Carbohydrate . . . . .13 g	
Dietary Fiber . . . . .1 g	
Sugars . . . . 9 g	
Protein . . . . 21 g	

Asian

Dressing

- **1/3** cup rice vinegar
- **1** Tbsp sesame oil
- **1** clove garlic, minced
- **2** tsp finely minced green onions
- **1/2** tsp minced ginger

Vegetables

- **1** cup sliced red pepper
- **1/2** cup thinly sliced celery
- **1/2** cup frozen peas, thawed and drained well
- **1/2** cup bean sprouts

Garnish:

- **1/4** cup roasted peanuts

Exchanges, Asian
3 Lean Meat   2 Vegetable

Calories 222	
Calories from Fat 98	
Total Fat . . . . .11 g	
Saturated Fat . . . . 2 g	
Cholesterol . . . . 36 mg	
Sodium . . . . 485 mg	
Total Carbohydrate . . . . . 9 g	
Dietary Fiber . . . . 3 g	
Sugars . . . . 3 g	
Protein . . . . 23 g	

Italian

Dressing

- **1/4** cup balsamic vinegar
- **1** Tbsp olive oil
- **1** Tbsp fat-free, reduced-sodium chicken broth
- **1** tsp minced fresh rosemary
- **1** clove garlic, minced

    Salt and pepper to taste

Vegetables

- **1** cup thinly-sliced jarred roasted red peppers
- **1/2** cup rehydrated sun-dried tomatoes
- **1** cup halved canned artichoke hearts in water, drained
- **2** Tbsp chopped black olives

Garnish:

- **2** tsp grated Parmesan cheese

French

Dressing

- **1/4** cup red or champagne vinegar
- **1** Tbsp olive oil
- **2** tsp Dijon mustard
- **2** tsp lemon juice
- **2** Tbsp minced shallots
- **1** clove garlic, minced

Vegetables

- **1** cup thinly sliced carrot
- **1** small tomato, seeded and diced
- **1/2** cup very thinly sliced red onion
- **1/2** cup peeled, seeded, and diced cucumber

Garnish:

- **1/4** cup crumbled Roquefort cheese

Serve on watercress leaves if desired.

Exchanges, Italian
3 Lean Meat 2 Vegetable

Calories	208
Calories from Fat	73
Total Fat	8 g
Saturated Fat	1 g
Cholesterol	37 mg
Sodium	718 mg
Total Carbohydrate	13 g
Dietary Fiber	2 g
Sugars	7 g
Protein	23 g

Exchanges, French
3 Lean Meat 2 Vegetable

Calories	195
Calories from Fat	75
Total Fat	8 g
Saturated Fat	2 g
Cholesterol	42 mg
Sodium	583 mg
Total Carbohydrate	8 g
Dietary Fiber	2 g
Sugars	5 g
Protein	22 g

Crunchy Shrimp and Broccoli Stir-Fry

Serving Size: 4 ounces, Total Servings: 4

The shrimp is coated in a bit of flour to give a crisp, crunchy coating without really frying the shrimp. The vegetables are just lightly stir-fried to keep each bright color. Hoisin sauce can be found in most grocery stores. It's a rich paste made from beans that really makes this sauce special.

1	lb large shrimp, peeled and deveined	1	cup sliced carrots
2	Tbsp all-purpose flour	1/2	cup sliced red pepper
1/4	tsp salt	1	cup broccoli florets
1/4	tsp pepper	1/4	cup fat-free, reduced-sodium chicken broth
2	tsp peanut oil	3	Tbsp lite soy sauce
2	tsp minced ginger	1/2	tsp sesame oil
2	cloves garlic, minced	1	Tbsp hoisin sauce
3	green onions, minced	1	Tbsp cornstarch

1 Combine the flour, salt, and pepper in a zippered plastic bag. Add the shrimp and toss to coat. Shake off excess flour and put the shrimp on a plate.

2 In a large wok or large heavy skillet, heat the peanut oil over medium-high heat. Add the shrimp and stir-fry for 3 minutes until shrimp turn pink and are slightly golden. Remove the shrimp from the pan and set aside.

3 Add the ginger, garlic, and green onions to the pan. Stir-fry for 1 minute. Add the carrots and stir-fry for 3 minutes. Add the red pepper and stir-fry for 3 minutes. Add the broccoli and stir-fry for 3 minutes.

4 Combine the broth, soy sauce, sesame oil, hoisin sauce, and cornstarch. Mix well. Add the sauce to the pan. Add back the shrimp. Cover and steam 1 minute. Toss well and serve.

PREPARATION
25 minutes

COOK
15 minutes

Exchanges
1/2 Starch
3 Very Lean Meat
1 Vegetable

Calories 166
   Calories from Fat 35
Total Fat . . . . 4 g
   Saturated Fat . . . . 1 g
Cholesterol . . . . 161 mg
Sodium . . . . 758 mg
Carbohydrate . . . . 13 g
   Dietary Fiber . . . . 2 g
   Sugars . . . . 5 g
Protein . . . . .19 g

Cioppino

Serving Size: 1 1/2 cups, Total Servings: 10

Cioppino is the pride of San Francisco. This dish was created by San Francisco's Italian immigrants and is a wonderful collection of seafood in a rich, heady tomato broth. Dip crusty whole-grain bread into a steaming bowl and there you have your meal.

2 Tbsp olive oil	1 (6-oz) can tomato paste
1 large onion, chopped	2 cups dry white wine
1 red pepper, chopped	1 tsp salt
1 green bell pepper, chopped	1/2 tsp pepper
3 cloves garlic, minced	1 lb rock cod, cut into 2-inch cubes
1/2 cup minced parsley	
1 tsp dried basil	1 lb shrimp, shelled and deveined
1 tsp dried oregano	12 fresh clams in shell, scrubbed
1 can (28-oz) plum tomatoes, coarsely chopped	

1 In a large kettle, heat the olive oil over medium heat. Add the onion and peppers and sauté for 5 minutes. Add the garlic, parsley, basil, and oregano. Stir in the tomatoes and their liquid, tomato paste, wine, salt, and pepper.

2 Bring to a boil, cover and reduce the heat, simmer for 1 hour. Uncover and boil over medium-low heat for 20 minutes.

3 Add the seafood. Cover and cook until clams open their shells and shrimp and rockfish are cooked through, about 15 minutes.

PREPARATION
20 minutes

COOK
1 hour and 40 minutes

Exchanges
3 Very Lean Meat
2 Vegetable

Calories 171
  Calories from Fat 35
Total Fat . . . . 4 g
  Saturated Fat . . . . 1 g
Cholesterol . . . . 98 mg
Sodium . . . . 489 mg
Carbohydrate . . . . 11 g
  Dietary Fiber . . . . 2 g
  Sugars . . . . 5 g
Protein . . . . 22 g

Seafood Kabobs Hawaiian

Serving Size: 2 (7-inch) kabobs or 1 (12-inch) kabob
Total Servings: 4

Kabobs are fun to eat! By simply changing the type of seafood and varying the fruits, you can come up with many interesting combinations. Soak wooden skewers in warm water for 15 minutes before putting the food on the skewer. This will prevent the skewer from burning on both ends while cooking.

1/2 cup dry sherry	1 large mango, peeled and cut into wedges
1 tsp sesame oil	1/2 papaya, peeled and cut into wedges
2 Tbsp grated fresh ginger	
2 Tbsp tamari soy sauce	1 large red pepper, seeded and cut into large squares
2 Tbsp pineapple juice concentrate	
1 lb fresh sea scallops or shrimp, peeled and deveined	

1 In a medium bowl, combine the sherry, sesame oil, ginger, soy sauce, and pineapple juice concentrate. Add the shrimp or scallops. Let the shellfish marinate for 30 minutes in the refrigerator.

2 Prepare an outside grill or oven broiler by placing the rack 6 inches from the heat source. Remove the shrimp or scallops from the marinade. Reserve the remaining marinade. Thread the shellfish onto wooden skewers and alternate them with the mango, papaya, and red pepper.

3 Place skewers on the grill and grill for about 5 minutes, turning and basting with the marinade.

PREPARATION
25 minutes, and
30 minutes marinating time

COOK
45 minutes

Exchanges
2 Very Lean Meat
1 1/2 Fruit

Calories 170
　Calories from Fat 16
Total Fat . . . . 2 g
　Saturated Fat . . . . 0 g
Cholesterol . . . . 95 mg
Sodium . . . . 429 mg
Carbohydrate . . . . 20 g
　Dietary Fiber . . . . .3 g
　Sugars . . . . .15 g
Protein . . . . .16 g

Stir-Fry Fish

Serving Size: about 4 ounces, Total Servings: 4

Most people would never dream of stir-frying chunks of fish. This very fast stir-fry brings out the best flavor in fish.

1 1/2 Tbsp canola oil	**1/2** cup fresh orange juice
1 lb rockfish, orange roughy, or bass, skin removed and cubed into 1 1/2-inch pieces	**2** tsp cornstarch or arrowroot
	1 tsp sesame oil
1 clove garlic, minced	**1** tsp rice vinegar
1 shallot, minced	**1** tsp lite soy sauce
1/2 cup chopped red pepper	
1/2 cup sliced celery	**Garnish:**
1 cup fresh snow peas, trimmed	Chopped green onions
1/2 cup water chestnuts	**2** cups cooked brown rice

1 In a wok or heavy skillet, over medium-high heat, heat 1 Tbsp of the oil. Add fish and stir-fry gently for 2–3 minutes. Remove the fish from the skillet and set aside.

2 Add the remaining 1/2 Tbsp oil and stir-fry the garlic and shallot for 1 minute. Add the red pepper, celery, snow peas, and water chestnuts. Cover the pan and let steam for 2 minutes.

3 Meanwhile, in a measuring cup or small dish, combine the orange juice, arrowroot, sesame oil, rice vinegar, and soy sauce. Add this mixture to the pan and cook until sauce thickens, about 1 minute. Garnish the dish with chopped green onions. Serve with cooked rice.

PREPARATION
20 minutes

COOK
10 minutes

Exchanges

2 Starch	2 Lean Meat
1 Vegetable	1/2 Fat

Calories 322
  Calories from Fat 87
Total Fat . . . . .10 g
  Saturated Fat . . . . .0 g
Cholesterol . . . . 47 mg
Sodium . . . . .152 mg
Carbohydrate . . . . .33 g
  Dietary Fiber . . . . 4 g
  Sugars . . . . 7 g
Protein . . . . 25 g

New Orleans Shrimp Creole

Serving Size: 1 cup, Total Servings: 6

All you need for dinner is in a bowl of this creole. You have all the healthy vegetables including the cancer-fighting tomatoes. Okra is also a nutritious vegetable, containing vitamins A and C. The okra also serves as a thickener; the liquid inside the okra will be drawn out and help make this creole hearty.

1/4 cup dry white wine

1 cup diced onions

1/2 cup diced celery

1 1/2 cups diced red pepper

1/2 cup diced green pepper

2 cloves garlic, minced

1 cup sliced okra

4 cups crushed canned tomatoes

1 Tbsp no-added-salt tomato paste

1 cup fat-free, reduced-sodium chicken broth

1/2 tsp cayenne pepper

1 tsp paprika

1/2 tsp celery seed

2 bay leaves

1 lb large shrimp, peeled and deveined

Salt and pepper to taste

1 In a large stockpot or kettle, heat the white wine over medium heat until it boils slightly.

2 Add the onions, celery, red and green pepper, and garlic and sauté for 10 minutes.

3 Add the okra, tomatoes, tomato paste, broth, cayenne pepper, paprika, celery seed, and bay leaves. Bring to a boil. Lower the heat and simmer for 45 minutes.

4 Add the shrimp and cook for 5–6 minutes more until the shrimp turn pink. Season with pepper and salt. Serve in bowls with cooked rice if desired.

PREPARATION
25 minutes

COOK
1 hour

Exchanges
1 Carbohydrate (equals 3 Vegetable)
2 Very Lean Meat
1 Vegetable

Calories 161
   Calories from Fat 10
Total Fat . . . . .1 g
   Saturated Fat . . . . .0 g
Cholesterol . . . . 107 mg
Sodium . . . . 670 mg
Carbohydrate . . . . .21 g
   Dietary Fiber . . . . .6 g
   Sugars . . . . .12 g
Protein . . . . .16 g

Shrimp Scampi

Serving Size: about 4 ounces, Total Servings: 4

This is for serious garlic lovers only! You will definitely get your cholesterol-reducing benefits from eating this much garlic. Sop up the pan juices with some crusty whole-grain bread.

1 lb large shrimp, peeled and deveined

2 Tbsp olive oil

2 tsp butter

6 cloves garlic, minced

3 Tbsp white wine

2 Tbsp minced parsley

Pinch crushed red pepper flakes

1 In a large heavy skillet over medium-high heat, heat the oil and butter. Add the garlic and sauté for 30 seconds. Add the white wine and raise the heat to high.

2 Add the shrimp and sauté for 3 minutes until shrimp turns pink. Add the parsley and red pepper flakes. Serve immediately.

PREPARATION
20 minutes

COOK
4 minutes

Exchanges
3 Very Lean Meat
1 1/2 Fat

Calories 163
　Calories from Fat 80
Total Fat . . . . 9 g
　Saturated Fat . . . . .3 g
Cholesterol . . . . .166 mg
Sodium . . . . .207 mg
Carbohydrate . . . . .2 g
　Dietary Fiber . . . . .0 g
　Sugars . . . . .1 g
Protein . . . . .18 g

Crispy Fish Filets

Serving Size: about 4 ounces, Total Servings: 4

No matter what we may know about good health, there are times we just crave the taste of fried foods. Fortunately with a good crumb mixture and the right technique, you can indeed enjoy fried fish. This recipe goes great with Sweet Potato Fries (see page 71).

Make sure you leave the fish for 20 minutes after rolling it in the crumbs. This will help the coating stick to the fish when you cook it.

Crumb mixture

1 cup soft bread crumbs	1/4 cup flour
2 Tbsp Parmesan cheese	Salt and pepper to taste
1 tsp dried oregano	2 egg substitutes
1/2 tsp dried basil	4 (4-oz) portions flounder, sole, orange roughy, or perch
1/2 tsp paprika	1 Tbsp canola oil
1/2 tsp garlic powder	
1/4 tsp onion powder	

1 Combine ingredients for the crumb mixture in a bowl.

2 Combine the flour with the salt and pepper.

3 In a medium bowl, beat the egg substitutes.

4 Dip each portion of fish first into the flour and shake off excess. Then dip into the egg. Roll each piece in the crumbs. Put the fish on a plate and refrigerator for 20 minutes.

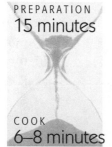

PREPARATION
15 minutes

COOK
6–8 minutes

5 Heat a large nonstick skillet over medium-high heat. Add the oil. Sauté the fish for 3-4 minutes per side until golden brown and fish is cooked through and opaque.

Exchanges
1 Starch
4 Very Lean Meat

Calories 223
    Calories from Fat 57
Total Fat . . . . 6 g
    Saturated Fat . . . . .1 g
Cholesterol . . . . 63 mg
Sodium . . . . 275 mg
Carbohydrate . . . . .12 g
    Dietary Fiber . . . . 0 g
    Sugars . . . . 1 g
Protein . . . . 28 g

Low-Fat Sauces for Fish

Serving Size: 2 Tbsp, Total Servings: 12 to 14

Tartar Sauce

Preparation time: 5 minutes

- **1** cup low-fat mayonnaise
- **2** Tbsp minced onion
- **1/4** cup minced dill pickle
- **1** Tbsp lemon juice
- **1** Tbsp mustard
- **2** tsp minced parsley

1 Mix together and serve with fish.

Cold Cucumber Sauce

Preparation time: 10 minutes
Chilling time: 30 minutes

- **1** cup plain low-fat yogurt
- **2** Tbsp reduced-fat sour cream
- **1/2** cup peeled, seeded, and diced cucumber
- **2** tsp apple cider vinegar
- **1** tsp minced dill
- **1** tsp minced parsley
- **1** tsp minced chives
- **1/2** tsp lemon zest

1 Mix all ingredients in a small bowl. Chill for 30 minutes. Use with cooked hot or cold salmon, turkey, or chicken.

Exchanges
1/2 Carbohydrate

Calories	36
Calories from Fat	13
Total Fat	1 g
Saturated Fat	0 g
Cholesterol	0 mg
Sodium	264 mg
Carbohydrate	6 g
Dietary Fiber	0 g
Sugars	4 g
Protein	0 g

Exchanges
Free food

Calories	14
Calories from Fat	4
Total Fat	0 g
Saturated Fat	0 g
Cholesterol	2 mg
Sodium	14 mg
Carbohydrate	2 g
Dietary Fiber	0 g
Sugars	1 g
Protein	1 g

Poultry

Poultry is economical, lean, and a good source of protein. Stick with lean cuts of poultry, specifically white meat chicken and turkey. Goose, duck, and the dark meat of chicken and turkey are higher in fat.

Nutrition Comparison

All portions are 3 1/2 ounces

Turkey	Calories	Fat
Breast w/o skin	135	1
Breast with skin	153	3
Leg w/o skin	159	4
Leg with skin	170	5
Wing w/o skin	163	3
Wing with skin	207	10
Ground	123	7

Chicken (broilers)	Calories	Fat
Breast w/o skin	165	4
Breast with skin	197	8
Leg w/o skin	191	8
Leg with skin	232	13
Wing w/o skin	203	8
Wing with skin	290	20
Ground	176	7

Duck	Calories	Fat
W/o skin	201	11
With skin	334	28

Cornish Hens	Calories	Fat
White meat	190	18
Dark meat	245	22

How to Buy

If you can, buy free-range, organic chickens. These chickens are not pent up in a small cage but are left to roam free. Their meat is more tender and less fatty. It's a real treat if it's available to you. Price-wise it really doesn't cost that much more than regular chicken and the taste is worth it.

We'll give you directions for purchasing chicken breasts, since the breast meat is lower in fat than the dark meat.

Try to buy chicken breast with the skin left on and bone removed. The skin will keep the chicken moist before you cook it and your final product will be much moister. Some fat is removed when the bone comes off.

Buy 4 1/4 to 4 1/2 ounces raw poultry with skin to get 3 ounces cooked. (Skin accounts for 1/4 to 1/2 ounce. Don't forget to remove it before or after cooking.)

Shop for poultry last on your trip around the supermarket. Check for freshness. You want a plump breast, a fresh smell, and no broken skin.

How to Store

Refrigerate poultry at 40°F as soon as you bring it home. Don't let it sit at room temperature more than 30 minutes. Cook poultry within 2 days of purchase.

Always freeze whatever chicken you think you won't use. First wrap it in butcher paper, then in zippered plastic freezer bags. Keep only about 6 months in the freezer. Don't defrost at room temperature. Thaw it in the refrigerator overnight.

Avoid defrosting and then refreezing chicken. The texture becomes very rubbery and distasteful.

Before Cooking

Wash the chicken in warm water and pat dry. Use clean knives and a clean cutting board. Many cooks keep a separate cutting board just for poultry. The jury is still out on whether a plastic or wooden board is better. A heavy plastic board cleans up beautifully in the dishwasher. Make sure you thoroughly clean knives, boards, and your hands after handling raw poultry. Leave the skin on up to when you are ready to cook to keep the meat moist.

Cooking

Chicken is done when no pink color remains. It is not vogue to eat pink chicken! Thoroughly cook the chicken.

Wild Rice Sun-dried Cherry Stuffed Chicken

Serving Size: about 4 ounces, 1/4 cup stuffing, Total Servings: 8

This dish is good for everyday, but is especially nice when company is coming. The sun-dried cherries provide extra vitamin C and the wild rice provides additional fiber to this dish.

4 whole chicken breasts, halved, skinned, and boned
   Salt and pepper

Stuffing

2 cups cooked wild rice	**1/2** cup minced celery
1 cup boiling water	**2** tsp minced fresh rosemary
1/2 cup sun-dried cherries	Salt and pepper to taste
1 Tbsp olive oil	**3/4** cup dry white wine
1 shallot, minced	Paprika

1 With a meat mallet, pound the breasts to 1/4-inch thickness. Sprinkle salt and pepper over each breast half. Set aside.

2 Prepare the rice according to package directions.

3 Meanwhile, in a small bowl, pour the boiling water over the cherries and let stand for 10 minutes. Drain.

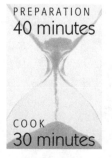

PREPARATION
40 minutes

COOK
30 minutes

4 In a small skillet over medium heat, heat the oil. Add the shallot and celery and sauté for 2 minutes. Add in the rosemary and sauté for 1 minute. Season with salt and pepper.

5 In a bowl, combine the cooked rice, cherries, and vegetable mixture.

6 To assemble the chicken: On a flat surface, spread the chicken breasts out for rolling. Use about 1/4 cup of stuffing for each chicken breast half and place on one end of the chicken breast. Roll the breast until it completely encases the stuffing. Tuck the end under. Secure with a toothpick. Repeat with all the breasts. Place the chicken breasts in a casserole dish and sprinkle paprika over each breast.

7 Pour the white wine in the casserole pan around the breasts. Bake at 350°F for 30–35 minutes, covered. Remove the cover during the last 5 minutes of cooking time to brown.

Exchanges

1/2 Starch	5 Very Lean Meat
1/2 Fruit	

Calories 257
   Calories from Fat 47
Total Fat . . . . 5 g
   Saturated Fat . . . . 1 g
Cholesterol . . . . 86 mg
Sodium . . . . 86 mg
Carbohydrate . . . . .16 g
   Dietary Fiber . . . . 1 g
   Sugars . . . . 5 g
Protein . . . . 33 g

Chicken with Tri-colored Peppers

Serving Size: 4 ounces chicken, Total Servings: 4

Stir-fried peppers have been made in our test kitchens for years. We added chicken breast and we have a complete meal. Shrimp is also great with this. Add more colored peppers if you can find them for a rainbow of color.

2 tsp canola oil

1 lb boneless, skinless chicken breasts, cut into 2-inch strips

1/2 cup diced onion

2 cloves garlic, minced

1 each small red, yellow, and green bell peppers, seeded and sliced into 1-inch strips

1/2 cup fat-free, reduced-sodium chicken broth

2 Tbsp lite soy sauce

1 Tbsp white wine (optional)

1/2 tsp sesame oil

2 tsp cornstarch

1 In a wok or heavy skillet over medium-high heat, heat the canola oil. Add the chicken and sauté for 2 minutes. Add the onion and garlic and sauté for 4–5 minutes more.

2 Remove the chicken and onion from the pan. Add the peppers and sauté for 5 minutes.

3 Combine the broth, soy sauce, white wine, sesame oil, and cornstarch in a measuring cup and mix well.

4 Add the sauce to the peppers. Add the chicken and onions back to the pan. Stir for 1–2 minutes until sauce has thickened.

PREPARATION
20 minutes

COOK
15 minutes

Exchanges

4 Very Lean Meat
2 Vegetable   1/2 Fat

Calories 204
    Calories from Fat 54
Total Fat . . . . 6 g
    Saturated Fat . . . . 1 g
Cholesterol . . . . 68 mg
Sodium . . . . 425 mg
Carbohydrate . . . . .10 g
    Dietary Fiber . . . . 2 g
    Sugars . . . . 5 g
Protein . . . . .27 g

Grilled Chicken Breasts with Fruit Salsa

Serving Size: about 4 ounces, Total Servings: 4

Fruit Salsa

2 cans (8 oz each) crushed pine-apple, packed in juice, drained

1 mango, peeled and cubed

1/2 papaya, peeled and cubed

2 Tbsp rice vinegar

1 Tbsp finely minced cilantro

1 Tbsp minced red pepper

2 whole chicken breasts, boned, skinned, halved (10 oz meat each)

2 tsp olive oil

Garnish: kiwi slices

1 In a medium bowl, combine salsa ingredients. Cover and refrigerate for 1 hour.

2 Preheat an oven broiler or outdoor grill. Brush the chicken breasts with the olive oil. Grill or broil the chicken about 7 minutes per side or until no pink remains.

3 To serve: Place fruit salsa on a plate using a few spoonfuls per person. Top with a cooked chicken breast. Garnish with kiwi slice.

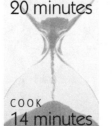

PREPARATION
20 minutes

COOK
14 minutes

Exchanges
4 Very Lean Meat
2 Fruit   1 Fat

Calories 305
 Calories from Fat 54
Total Fat . . . . 6 g
 Saturated Fat . . . . 2 g
Cholesterol . . . . 85 mg
Sodium . . . . 79 mg
Carbohydrate . . . . 30 g
 Dietary Fiber . . . . 3 g
 Sugars . . . . 25 g
Protein . . . . 32 g

Chicken Salad in 64+ Ways

Serving Size: about 4 ounces, Total Servings: 4

You can have chicken salad every day for a month and not repeat the exact flavors. This system is so much fun, you might invent yet another 64 ways to make a perennial favorite.

Master Recipe

Chicken

1 lb boneless, skinless chicken breasts

Water to cover

2 whole peppercorns

1 small onion, sliced

Vegetables

3 stalks celery, diced

1 small onion, minced

1 small red pepper, diced

Dressing

3/4 cup low-fat mayonnaise

2 Tbsp low-fat sour cream

Salt and pepper to taste

1 In a skillet, add the chicken, water to cover, peppercorns, and sliced onion. Bring to a boil, lower the heat to simmer, cover, and simmer for 10 minutes until chicken is cooked through. Remove chicken using a slotted spoon and put on a plate to cool. When cool enough to handle, cut the chicken into 2-inch cubes.

2 Mix the dressing ingredients.

3 Add the celery, onion, and red pepper to the chicken. Add the dressing and mix well. Refrigerate for 1/2 hour.

PREPARATION
20 minutes

COOK
10 minutes

Exchanges, Master Recipe

1 Carbohydrate
4 Very Lean Meat
1/2 Fat

Calories 232
   Calories from Fat 59
Total Fat . . . . 7 g
   Saturated Fat . . . . 1 g
Cholesterol . . . . 71 mg
Sodium . . . . 513 mg
Carbohydrate . . . . .16 g
   Dietary Fiber . . . . 1 g
   Sugars . . . . 11 g
Protein . . . . 26 g

Variations

List A: Choose a different dressing:

1. 1/4 cup olive oil mixed with 3 Tbsp lemon juice
2. 1/4 cup olive oil mixed with 3 Tbsp red wine vinegar
3. 1/4 cup olive oil mixed with 3 Tbsp balsamic vinegar
4. Any of the above, heated

List B: Choose a different vegetable filling:

1. 1/4 cup green onions and 1/2 cup sliced jarred roasted red pepper
2. 1 cup sliced canned artichoke hearts and 1/2 cup diced red onion
3. 1 cup halved cherry tomatoes and 2 Tbsp capers
4. 1 cup rehydrated sun-dried tomatoes and 2 Tbsp sliced black olives

List C: Add an herb:

1. 1 Tbsp minced thyme
2. 1 Tbsp minced basil
3. 1/2 tsp red pepper flakes
4. 1 Tbsp minced tarragon

Follow the master recipe, substituting a dressing from list A for the mayonnaise and sour cream dressing, a vegetable filling from List B for the celery, onion, and red pepper, and add an herb of choice from List C. Make many variations by combining different ingredients, i.e.
A2 + B3 + C2 or A1 + B4 + C3 and so on!

Exchanges, Chicken Salad in 64 Ways, Olive Oil & Balsamic Variation

4 Very Lean Meat
1 Vegetable
2 Fat

Calories	264
Calories from Fat	136
Total Fat	15 g
Saturated Fat	4 g
Cholesterol	68 mg
Sodium	88 mg
Carbohydrate	6 g
Dietary Fiber	1 g
Sugars	3 g
Protein	26 g

Oriental Turkey Salad

Serving Size: about 4 ounces turkey, Total Servings: 4

Here is a creative way to use leftover cooked turkey or chicken. Even if your turkey is a bit dried out, it doesn't matter; this dressing will revive the flavor. Soba noodles are made from buckwheat and are a very healthy food. Throughout the Asian countries you'll find these noodles and fortunately you can get soba noodles in most Asian grocery stores and regular supermarkets throughout the United States.

2 cups leftover cooked turkey, sliced into 2-inch strips, or 1 lb turkey filets, cooked and sliced into 2-inch strips

2 cups sliced celery

1 cup fresh snow peas, trimmed

1/2 cup diced red pepper

1/2 cup minced green onions

1 cup cooked soba noodles (or any other noodle)

Dressing

6 Tbsp rice vinegar

2 tsp sesame oil

1 tsp honey

2 tsp dry sherry or white wine

2 cloves garlic, minced

Fresh ground pepper and salt to taste

4 large romaine lettuce leaves

2 Tbsp toasted sesame seeds

1 In a large salad bowl, toss the turkey with the vegetables and soba noodles.

2 In a measuring cup or small bowl, whisk together the dressing ingredients.

3 Pour dressing over salad.

PREPARATION
25 minutes

4 To serve, line plates with lettuce, top with salad, and garnish with toasted sesame seeds.

Exchanges
1/2 Carbohydrate
3 Lean Meat
1 Vegetable

Calories 233
   Calories from Fat 74
Total Fat . . . . 8 g
   Saturated Fat . . . . .1 g
Cholesterol . . . . 54 mg
Sodium . . . . .126 mg
Carbohydrate . . . . 16 g
   Dietary Fiber . . . . .3 g
   Sugars . . . . .5 g
Protein . . . . 24 g

Meats

It's on to the meat case. Meat does add fat, saturated fat, and cholesterol to the diet. But meats are sources of high-quality, complete protein, good sources of some B vitamins (niacin, thiamin, B6, and B12), and zinc. Meats are also good sources of iron, and it's heme iron, which is better absorbed than the nonheme iron found in plant foods. As long as you choose lean cuts and vary your meat consumption with seafood and poultry, you don't have to give up meat as part of your healthy food plan.

Fortunately today, butchers are more careful about trimming the fat from the meat. To ensure you are getting the leanest cuts here is what you need to do.

A visual check

Look at the meat to see the extent of marbling. Marbling is the white streaks of fat running through the meat. Although marbling makes a cut of meat more tender it also raises its fat content.

Understand the grading process

Meat is graded by the government. Grade depends on the amount of marbling.

Prime: The most expensive cut, the most tender, but also the highest in fat.

Choice: Less fatty than prime, but inspect carefully. The fat content can still be quite high.

Select: The leanest of the cuts, although you will have to use cooking methods that tenderize the meat.

You can also select meat according to its name. The terms "loin" or "round" indicate a cut that is lean.

When looking at ground meat products, look for percentages rather than the terminology of lean or extra lean. The higher the percentage of lean, the lower in fat the product will be. If you don't see what you need that is already ground, ask the butcher to take a round steak and grind it for you. Ground round will be the leanest cut, followed by ground sirloin, ground chuck, and then regular ground beef.

Buying Meat

Be sure to check the sell date of the product. You'll want to cook the meat before the sell date if you aren't planning on freezing it.

Good quality meat will have a bright red color. Avoid meat that has a purplish or brown color. It may indicate the meat has been exposed to air and was not packaged properly.

Pork and lamb can provide interesting alternatives to beef. With pork, also be sure to buy the leanest cuts: loin roast, tenderloin, loin chop, rib roast, and rib chop. Buy pork that is pink, not gray. A grayish tinge means the pork is past its prime. Lamb should be bright pink, not bright red, which may indicate the lamb is old and tough.

Precooked hams can also be enjoyed, since they can be up to 95% fat free. However, hams can be very high in sodium and you should figure that in your daily allotment of sodium. If you want bacon, stick with Canadian bacon, which is taken from the loin area and is much leaner than traditional bacon.

How Much?

The ounces of meat specified in your meal plan are for cooked quantities. When you purchase a piece of meat, estimate the amount of raw meat you need to buy.

Raw meat with no bone: 4 oz raw = 3 oz cooked
Raw meat with bone: 5 oz raw = 3 oz cooked

Think about how many people you are feeding, how much they will each eat (or should eat), what quantity you will lose in cooking, and how much you want for leftovers. That's your number. Write this amount by the item on your shopping list or do your calculation at the meat counter.

Marinated Steak Kabobs

Serving Size: 4 ounces meat, Total Servings: 4

What kind of summer would it be without some form of kabob on the grill? Sirloin steak is a good choice for making kabobs. It has just the right fat content to ensure a flavorful meat, yet lean enough to include on a low-fat eating plan.

1/4 cup lite soy sauce

1 Tbsp honey

2 Tbsp dry sherry

1 tsp orange zest

1 Tbsp canola oil

1 lb sirloin steak, trimmed of any fat and cut into 1 1/2-inch cubes

1 large green pepper, seeded and cut into 1-inch squares

1 large red pepper, seeded and cut into 1-inch squares

1 Combine the soy sauce, honey, sherry, zest, and oil in a zippered plastic bag. Add the beef and close the bag. Refrigerate for 2 hours or overnight.

2 Drain marinade. Soak wooden skewers in a pan of warm water for 30 minutes. Thread the steak and peppers alternately onto skewers.

3 Prepare an oven broiler or outdoor grill with the rack set 4 inches from the heat source. Grill on each side over medium heat for a total of about 10 minutes, or until desired degree of doneness.

PREPARATION
20 minutes, and
2 hours or more marinating time

COOK
10 minutes

Exchanges
3 Lean Meat
2 Vegetable

Calories 194
   Calories from Fat 62
Total Fat . . . . 7 g
   Saturated Fat . . . . 2 g
Cholesterol . . . . 64 mg
Sodium . . . . 354 mg
Carbohydrate . . . . 9 g
   Dietary Fiber . . . . 2 g
   Sugars . . . . 5 g
Protein . . . . 23 g

Chinese Stir-Fried Beef with Ginger

Serving Size: 4 ounces beef, Total Servings: 4

Ginger is one of those spices that tastes so much better when you use it fresh. If for any reason you can't get it, substitute 2 tsp ground ginger. The peel of fresh ginger is so paper thin you can just mince the ginger without peeling it. Add any other vegetables such as broccoli, bean sprouts, bok choy, or carrots in place of the vegetables listed here.

Beef Mixture

1 lb lean round steak, cut into 2-inch strips

2 Tbsp lite soy sauce

1 tsp sesame oil

2 Tbsp dry sherry

Dash crushed red pepper flakes

1 tsp peanut or canola oil

1 Tbsp minced ginger

2 cloves garlic, minced

1 small onion, thinly sliced

1 small red pepper, seeded and cut into 1-inch strips

1 cup snow peas, trimmed

1 In a medium bowl, combine the steak, soy sauce, sesame oil, sherry, and crushed red pepper flakes. Cover and refrigerate for 1 hour.

2 In a wok or heavy skillet, heat the canola or peanut oil. Add the beef and stir-fry for about 5–6 minutes until beef loses its pinkness. Remove the beef from the wok and set aside.

3 Add the ginger and garlic to the pan and stir-fry for 1 minute. Add the onion and stir-fry for 1 minute. Add the red pepper and stir-fry for 2 minutes. Add the snow peas and stir-fry for 2 minutes.

4 Add the beef back to the wok and heat for 1 minute. Serve with additional lite soy sauce if desired.

PREPARATION
20 minutes, and
1 hour marinating time

COOK
15 minutes

Exchanges

3 Lean Meat   1 Vegetable

Calories 179
    Calories from Fat 63
Total Fat . . . . .7 g
    Saturated Fat . . . . .2 g
Cholesterol . . . . .58 mg
Sodium . . . . .235 mg
Carbohydrate . . . . .7 g
    Dietary Fiber . . . . .2 g
    Sugars . . . . .4 g
Protein . . . . .20 g

Spiced Lamb Stew

Serving Size: 4 ounces lamb, Total Servings: 4

You'll want to prepare this once the weather gets chilly. It makes a nice change from beef stew. Sweet potatoes and carrots pack plenty of vitamin A.

1 tsp cinnamon

1/2 tsp ground coriander

1/4 tsp ground cinnamon

1/4 tsp ground ginger

1/8 tsp salt

1/4 tsp black pepper

1 lb lean lamb, cut into 1-inch cubes

2 carrots, sliced diagonally

1 small sweet potato, cut into 1-inch cubes

1 green pepper, cut into 2-inch squares

1 clove garlic, minced

1/4 cup flour

3 cups fat-free, reduced-sodium chicken broth

Dash hot sauce

2 Tbsp minced parsley

1 Combine the cinnamon, coriander, cinnamon, ginger, salt, and pepper. Coat the lamb chunks with the spice mixture.

2 In a large skillet or Dutch oven sprayed with nonstick spray, sauté the lamb pieces for 5 minutes. Add the carrots, sweet potato, green pepper, and garlic and sauté for 5 minutes. Sprinkle the stew with flour until well coated. Add the broth and bring to a boil.

3 Lower the heat and simmer for 20–25 minutes until lamb is tender and vegetables are cooked through. Add the hot sauce and parsley.

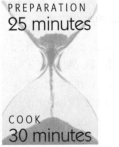

PREPARATION
25 minutes

COOK
30 minutes

Exchanges
1 Starch
3 Lean Meat
1 Vegetable

Calories 287
    Calories from Fat 78
Total Fat . . . . 9 g
    Saturated Fat . . . . 3 g
Cholesterol . . . . 81 mg
Sodium . . . . 524 mg
Carbohydrate . . . . 21 g
    Dietary Fiber . . . . 3 g
    Sugars . . . . 8 g
Protein . . . . 30 g

Eggs

Eggs are an excellent source of protein, providing about 10% of your total protein needs per day, 25% of the daily requirement for vitamin B12, and moderate amounts of folic acid and minerals. They have only about 5 grams total fat and only 1 gram of that fat is saturated.

We know, your next question is about cholesterol.

Research has shown that saturated fat is far more likely to raise a person's blood cholesterol levels than dietary cholesterol. Otherwise healthy adults can eat up to 3-4 eggs per week.

If you want to limit your consumption of cholesterol, in cooking you can often use a combination of whole eggs and egg whites, keeping the cholesterol down and the flavor up. Also, the quality of egg substitutes has come a long way.

Here is a nutritional comparison of yolks versus whites:

	Yolk	White	Whole
Calories	58	17	75
Protein (g)	2	4	6
Saturated fat (g)	1.5	0	1.5
Cholesterol (mg)	213	0	213
Vitamin A (IU)	318	0	318
Vitamin B12 (mcg)	0.4	0.1	0.5
Folic acid (mcg)	23	1	24

How to Buy

The shell color doesn't indicate the nutritional value, only the breed of hen. Eggs are graded AA, A, and B. This grading system refers to the exterior and interior quality of the egg. Most eggs sold in supermarkets will be of A quality.

Inspect eggs before buying them. Don't buy eggs with cracks. Buy only what you will use. Consider purchasing half cartons or using egg substitutes if you only use eggs on occasion.

Storing

Eggs are perishable and should be stored carefully. The manufacturer of your refrigerator thought egg cups on the inside of your refrigerator door was a good idea, but if you store them there, the temperature of the eggs will change every time you open the refrigerator.

Keep eggs in their original carton, pointed side down. Put the carton towards the back of the refrigerator where the temperature is coldest. Use up eggs within 3-4 weeks after bringing them home. Don't leave eggs at room temperature longer than 2 hours.

Cooking with Eggs

Freshness Test. One of the first science experiments you probably remember from your grade school days still applies. Fill a bowl full of water. Add the egg. A fresh egg will sink to the bottom. A stale egg will float; don't use it.

Always Cook. Be safe: Don't serve dishes made with raw eggs such as Caesar salads, mousses, or eggnog, unless pasteurized.

Beating Eggs. Often recipes will call for beaten eggs. A smart way to get the egg nutrients without too much cholesterol is to use egg whites or a combination of whole eggs and whites. An omelette, for example, can be made with 1 egg and 2 beaten egg whites folded in. Your omelette will be nice and full, as if it had been made with 3 whole eggs. Here is the proper procedure for beating egg whites:

1. Let eggs (uncracked) sit on the counter at room temperature for 15 minutes.

2. Use a bowl that is very clean and free of grease. Use glass, porcelain, or stainless steel rather than plastic, which can harbor odors and grease.

3. Using either a balloon whisk or hand-held electric mixer, whip the egg whites until they form stiff, moist peaks.

4. Once they're whipped, don't delay—add to your recipe.

Egg-citing Eggs!

* To scrambled eggs: Add a few slices of roasted red peppers from the jar and 1 tsp of capers for a Mediterranean flavor.

* Add bean sprouts and fresh snow peas to an omelette. Drizzle lite soy sauce on the top of the omelette.

* Make a zesty egg salad. To 1 chopped egg and 3 chopped egg whites, fold in 1/3 cup low-fat plain yogurt, 2 tsp Dijon mustard, 1/4 tsp garlic powder, 2 Tbsp minced red onion, 2 Tbsp minced celery, and 2 Tbsp minced red pepper.

* Make a lower-fat, lower-calorie Egg McMuffin: Poach 1 egg. Put 1 ounce Canadian bacon on a toasted whole-wheat English muffin. Top with egg and 1 Tbsp low-fat cheddar cheese. Put under the broiler for 1 minute until cheese melts. Serve open-face.

Meat and Meat Substitutes

	Exchange/ Serving	Calories	Protein (g)	Total Fat (g)	Sat. Fat (g)	Cholesterol (mg)
VERY LEAN						
Meat						
Beef, chipped, dried (sodium)	1 oz	47	8	1	0.5	26
Buffalo	1 oz	40	8	0.5	0.5	23
Chicken, white meat, no skin	1 oz	49	9	1.5	0.5	24
Cornish hen, no skin	1 oz	38	7	1	0.5	30
Sausage, hard, < 1 gm fat/oz	1 oz	35	4	1	0.5	12
Turkey, white meat, no skin	1 oz	44	8	1	0.5	20
Turkey ham	1 oz	36	5	1.5	0.5	16
Venison	1 oz	45	8	1	0.5	32
Fish						
Cod	1 oz	30	6	0	0	16
Flounder	1 oz	33	7	0.5	0	19
Haddock	1 oz	32	7	0.5	0	21
Halibut	1 oz	40	8	1	0	12
Trout	1 oz	54	8	2.5	0.5	21
Tuna	1 oz	52	8	2	0.5	14
Tuna, canned, water pack, drained	1 oz	33	7	0.5	0	9
Shellfish						
Clams, canned, drained	1 oz	42	7	0.5	0	19
Clams, fresh, steamed	1 oz	42	7	0.5	0	19
Crab, canned, drained	1 oz	28	6	0.5	0	26
Crab, steamed	1 oz	29	6	0.5	0	28
Imitation shellfish	1 oz	29	3	0.5	0	6
Lobster, steamed	1 oz	28	6	0	0	20
Scallops, steamed	1 oz	32	7	0.5	0	15
Shrimp, canned, drained	1 oz	34	7	0.5	0	50
Shrimp, fresh	1 oz	28	6	0.5	0	56
Cheese						
Cheese, fat-free	1 oz	37	6	0	0	0
Cottage cheese, dry	1/4 cup	31	6	0	0	2
Cottage cheese, nonfat	1/4 cup	35	6	0	0	5
Cottage cheese, low-fat (2%)	1/4 cup	50	8	1	0.5	5

(continued)

Meat and Meat Substitutes

	Exchange/ Serving	Calories	Protein (g)	Total Fat (g)	Sat. Fat (g)	Cholesterol (mg)
Other						
Egg whites	2	34	7	0	0	0
Egg substitute	1/4 cup	35	6	0	0	0
Hot dog, < 1 gm fat/oz (sodium)	1 oz	30	4	1	0.5	11
Kidney, beef, simmered	1 oz	41	7	1	0.5	110

LEAN

	Exchange/ Serving	Calories	Protein (g)	Total Fat (g)	Sat. Fat (g)	Cholesterol (mg)
Beef						
Chuck/blade pot roast, cooked	1 oz	62	9	2.5	1	29
Cubed steak, cooked	1 oz	58	9	2	0.5	27
Flank steak, broiled, lean	1 oz	59	8	3	1	19
Ground round	1 oz	56	10	1.5	0.5	26
Porterhouse, broiled	1 oz	62	8	3	1	23
Rib roast, lean, roasted	1 oz	65	8	3.5	1.5	23
Round steak, broiled, lean	1 oz	55	8	2.5	1	23
Rump roast, lean, braised	1 oz	60	9	2.5	1	27
Sirloin	1 oz	54	9	2	1	25
T-bone, broiled	1 oz	61	8	3	1	23
Tenderloin, broiled, lean	1 oz	67	8	3.5	1.5	24
Pork						
Canadian bacon, grilled (sodium)	1 oz	53	7	2.5	1	16
Ham, boiled lean, sandwich type	1 oz	46	5	2.5	1	15
Ham, canned (fully cooked)	1 oz	48	6	2.5	1	12
Ham, cured, roasted	1 oz	45	7	1.5	0.5	16
Ham, fresh (pork leg), baked	1 oz	60	8	3	1	27
Pork tenderloin, cooked	1 oz	47	8	1.5	0.5	23
Pork loin, roast/chop, center cut, roasted	1 oz	60	8	2.5	1	23
Lamb						
Lamb leg, sirloin, roasted, lean	1 oz	58	8	2.5	1	26
Lamb loin, roast/chop, roasted	1 oz	57	8	3	1	25
Poultry						
Chicken, dark meat, no skin	1 oz	58	8	3	1	26
Chicken, light meat with skin, roasted	1 oz	63	8	3	1	24

(continued)

Meat and Meat Substitutes

	Exchange/ Serving	Calories	Protein (g)	Total Fat (g)	Sat. Fat (g)	Cholesterol (mg)
Poultry (cont'd)						
Duck, domestic, meat only, roasted	1 oz	57	7	3	1	25
Goose, roasted	1 oz	68	8	3.5	1.5	27
Turkey, dark meat, no skin	1 oz	53	8	2	0.5	24
Turkey pastrami, < 3 g fat/oz	1 oz	40	5	2	0.5	15
Fish						
Catfish filet	1 oz	43	5	2.5	0.5	18
Herring, smoked	1 oz	62	7	3.5	1	23
Oysters, medium	6	58	6	2	0.5	44
Salmon, filet broiled/baked	1 oz	61	8	3	0.5	25
Salmon, canned in water, drained	1 oz	40	6	1.5	0.5	11
Sardines, oil-pack, drained	2	50	6	2.5	0.5	34
Tuna, canned in oil, drained	1 oz	56	8	2.5	0.5	5
Cheese						
Cheddar/colby, low-fat	1 oz	49	7	2	1	6
Cottage, 4.5%	1/4 cup	54	6	2.5	1.5	8
Mozzarella, light	1 oz	65	8	3	2	15
Parmesan, grated	2 Tbsp	46	4	3	2	8
Organ meats						
Heart, beef, simmered	1 oz	50	8	1.5	0.5	55
Liver, beef, braised	1 oz	46	7	1.5	0.5	110
Liver, chicken, simmered	1 oz	45	7	1.5	0.5	180

MEDIUM-FAT

	Exchange/ Serving	Calories	Protein (g)	Total Fat (g)	Sat. Fat (g)	Cholesterol (mg)
Beef						
Corned brisket, cooked	1 oz	72	5	5.5	2	28
Ground, extra lean, broiled	1 oz	73	7	4.5	2	24
Ground, lean, broiled	1 oz	78	7	5.5	2	25
Ground, regular, broiled	1 oz	82	7	6	2.5	26
Prime rib, roasted	1 oz	83	8	5.5	2.5	23
Shortribs	1 oz	83	9	5	2	26
Lamb						
Ground	1 oz	80	7	5.5	2.5	28
Rib, roast	1 oz	67	8	3.5	1.5	26

(continued)

Meat and Meat Substitutes

	Exchange/ Serving	Calories	Protein (g)	Total Fat (g)	Sat. Fat (g)	Cholesterol (mg)
Pork						
Boston blade, roasted	1 oz	66	7	4	1.5	24
Poultry						
Chicken, dark meat with skin, roasted	1 oz	72	7	4.5	1	26
Chicken, fried, flour-coated	1 oz	76	8	4	1	26
Turkey, ground	1 oz	67	8	3.5	1	29
Cheese						
Feta	1 oz	74	4	6	4	25
Mozzarella, part skim	1 oz	72	7	4.5	3	16
Ricotta, part skim	1/4 cup	86	7	5	3	19
Soy						
Tempeh	1/4 cup	83	8	3	0.5	0
Tofu	1/2 cup	88	9	5.5	1	0
Other						
Egg	1	74	6	5	1.5	213
Fish, fried, breaded	1 oz	65	5	4	1	23

HIGH-FAT

These items are high in saturated fat, cholesterol, and calories and may raise blood cholesterol levels if eaten on a regular basis.

	Exchange/ Serving	Calories	Protein (g)	Total Fat (g)	Sat. Fat (g)	Cholesterol (mg)
Meat						
Bacon, fried, drained	3 slices (20 slices/lb)	105	5	9	3	15
Bologna, beef and pork	1 oz	89	3	8	3	16
Bratwurst, pork, cooked	1 oz	85	4	7.5	2.5	17
Hot dog, turkey (sodium)	1 frank (10/lb)	102	6	8	2.5	48
Knockwurst	1 oz	87	3	8	3	16
Pickle and pimiento loaf	1 oz	74	3	6	2	10
Pork, ground	1 oz	84	7	6	2	27
Pork sausage, pattie/link, cooked	1 oz	105	6	9	3	24
Pork spareribs, braised	1 oz	113	8	8.5	3	35
Sausage, smoked	1 oz	96	4	8.5	3	20

(continued)

Meat and Meat Substitutes

	Exchange/ Serving	Calories	Protein (g)	Total Fat (g)	Sat. Fat (g)	Cholesterol (mg)
Cheese						
American, processed (sodium)	1 oz	106	6	9	5.5	27
Cheddar	1 oz	114	7	9.5	6	30
Monterey jack	1 oz	106	7	8.5	5.5	27
Swiss	1 oz	107	8	8	5	26
1 HIGH-FAT MEAT + 1 FAT						
Hot dog, beef and pork (sodium)	1 frank (10/lb)	144	5	13	5	22
Peanut butter	2 Tbsp	188	7	16 (7.5 g mono, 4.5 g poly)	3	0

All meats are trimmed of fat and cooked, unless noted.
(sodium) = 400 mg or more of sodium per exchange.

RECIPES

FATS

✈ Herbed Avocado Dressing _____ 241

✈ Whole-Wheat Flax Loaf _____ 243

✈ New Waldorf Salad _____ 246

✈ Chinese Chicken with Cashews _____ 247

LOWER-FAT PARTY FOODS

Sun-Dried Tomato Spread _____ 248

Smoky Cheese Dip _____ 249

Hot Artichoke Dip _____ 250

Hummus _____ 251

Creamy Spinach Dip _____ 252

Potato Skin Bar _____ 253

Open-Faced Mini Bagel Bar

    Veggie Sandwich _____ 254

    Turkey Chutney Sandwiches _____ 255

    Tomato Pizza Bagels _____ 255

Low-Fat Buffalo Wings _____ 256

The fat group includes foods that are all or mostly fat. A serving or exchange of fat has 5 grams of fat and 45 calories. As you saw in Focus on Fats (p. 159), fats are divided into three main categories: monounsaturated, polyunsaturated, and saturated. That makes it easier to choose healthy fats.

THE REALLY GOOD FATS: MONOUNSATURATED

- Avocado
- Oils (canola, olive, peanut)
- Olives
- Nuts
- Peanut butter

Olive and canola oil are the highest in monounsaturated fat, and they're both Nutrition Superstars. But don't forget that fat is fat when it comes to calories. Oils and foods with monounsaturated fat are no lower in calories than the less-healthy oils.

Max Out on Monos

- Stock canola and olive oil instead of poly-unsaturated oils. Use these oils to sauté, cook, and bake. Use canola oil to bake; olive oil has too heavy a taste for baked goods. Keep oils stored in a cool dry place or in the refrigerator for best freshness. Remove from the refrigerator 15 minutes before preparing your recipe to allow the oil to decloud.

- Olive oil is renowned for its taste. You can select olive oil according to its grade. You need only purchase an extra virgin (oil from the first pressing of the olives). This is the best-tasting of the olive oils and has the lowest acidity and richest flavor.

- Another way to go is to purchase the flavored oils. Oils can be flavored with lemon, garlic, herbs, and spices. Just a dab on foods can give them great flavor.

- Buy salad dressing made with canola or olive oil, and canola-based margarine and mayonnaise.

- Make your own salad dressing with canola or olive oil.

- Toss a few nuts, ground flax seeds, or sesame seeds on salads, casseroles, cereals, or stir-fries.

- Use a slice or two of avocado on a salad or sandwich or to garnish a casserole. Enjoy guacamole on occasion with baked or fat-free tortilla chips.

- Enjoy a few olives on the side of a sandwich, tossed on a salad, or on a relish tray.

POLYUNSATURATED FATS

- Oils (corn, safflower, sunflower, cottonseed, soybean, and "vegetable oil")

- Margarine

- Mayonnaise

Polyunsaturated oils are commonly used in commercial food preparation of crackers, cookies, and other foods that contain fat.

THE BAD GUYS: SATURATED FATS

- Butter
- Cream cheese
- Sour cream
- Bacon

The message is loud and clear: Eat less saturated fat. Choose low-fat cream cheese, and low-fat or fat-free sour cream. Read the labels of processed foods. Check for tropical oils (coconut, palm oils) and see how far down on the ingredient list they fall. The further down, the better. You'll also want to eat less of the related fats: hydrogenated and trans.

Hydrogenated Fat

Hydrogenated fats are unsaturated fats that are processed, or "hydrogenated," to make them more solid at room temperature. The process of hydrogenation makes a fat more saturated. Stick margarine is made by hydrogenating liquid vegetable oil.

Trans Fats

Trans fats are formed in the process of hydrogenating fats. Although trans fats are unsaturated, their effects appear similar to saturated fats in that they seem to raise blood cholesterol levels.

The majority of trans fats come from processed foods that have partially-hydrogenated oils, such as commercially-prepared snacks, crackers, cookies, cakes, fried foods, and some margarines. Partially-hydrogenated oils are used in processed foods because they help food stay fresh longer and have a better texture. Trans fats also occur naturally in small amounts in meats and dairy products. Trans fats from all sources provide only 2 to 4% of the total fat and calories in the American diet.

Taper Off Trans and Hydrogenated Fats

Because of the potential negative effects of trans fats, it's a good idea to taper off trans fats.

- Reduce total fat intake. This helps lower your intake of both saturated and trans fats.

- Read the ingredient label for foods that contain hydrogenated or partially-hydrogenated fat and minimize how many of these foods you buy. (The amount of trans fats in a food is not required on the Nutrition Facts at the moment. The FDA is currently considering a proposed rule for labeling of trans fats.)

- Choose margarine that is low in trans fats (the soft tub magarines), or one that is labeled trans fat-free.

- Try reduced-fat, low-fat, fat-free, and trans fat–free versions of foods you often eat.

- In restaurants, minimize the amount of fried foods you eat as these likely contain some trans fats.

REPLACING FAT

Why do chefs love to load on the butter?
Why do French fries and ice cream taste so good?
The answer is simple: Fat.

Fat makes food taste good! Fat carries flavor and provides "mouthfeel." Fats coat the taste buds with taste sensations. Fat also helps you feel full and satisfied. Fats give and maintain moistness in foods like baked goods. They help blend ingredients, which is important for mayonnaise and salad dressings.

But many people want to eat less fat. To address this demand, food manufacturers make some foods with fat replacers.

The majority of fat replacers used today are carbohydrate-based. When fat is taken out and these fat replacers are put in, the fat content is lower, but often the carbohydrate content increases. This is something you need to factor in to your carbohydrate count.

Foods like ice cream, sour cream, cream cheese, salad dressing, potato chips, and margarine are available in lower-fat forms. You might have to try several before you find one that tastes good to you.

Remember, these products are not calorie-free or carbohydrate-free. Read the Nutrition Facts to check the grams of carbohydrate.

BUTTER VS. MARGARINE: WHAT'S BEST

Today, there are enough butters, margarines, blends, and spreads to keep you reading until you can't see straight.

Butter

Butter, because it's an animal product, contains cholesterol and saturated fat. But the amount per teaspoon is minimal: 2 milligrams of saturated fat and 10 milligrams of cholesterol.

If your blood fats are in a good range, and you prefer the taste of butter and you use it sparingly, then use butter. You could also opt for a margarine-butter blend or a light tub butter. Either of these choices is lower in cholesterol and saturated fat than stick butter.

Margarine

Margarine is made from unsaturated vegetable oil, so it has no cholesterol. That's good. But margarine is hydrogenated, meaning some unsaturated fat is made saturated. There is also the concern that hydrogenation adds trans fats to margarine that aren't present in butter.

If you have a big problem with your blood cholesterol and LDL cholesterol levels, then opt for margarine. Select a tub margarine. You might want to keep a liquid squeeze margarine around for some purposes.

Today there are margarines on the market that are canola-oil based or trans-free, and these are healthier choices. There are even margarines and salad dressings made with certain fatty acids that actually lower LDL cholesterol if used regularly. Try several brands, find products that meet the needs of both your palate and your health.

Whichever you choose, remember butter and margarine are both fat, and fat is calories. If you can cut down on the amount of butter or margarine you use, you'll eat less total fat and less saturated fat. Also, think of using canola or olive oil rather than margarine or butter when the use fits.

Take advantage of the food label to take the guess work and confusion out of your decision. Most of them list total fat, cholesterol, and saturated fat. Some list polyunsaturated and monounsaturated fat.

Avocado

Avocados are a good source of monounsaturated fat and have 1 gram of fiber per serving. Don't forget, though, they are mainly fat and therefore contain a hefty number of calories.

How to Buy: Avocados are available year-round in most parts of the country. The two most widely marketed avocados are the black, pebbly-skinned Haas and the green, smooth-skinned Fuerte. Select unblemished avocados that yield to slight pressure.

How to Store: Put unripe avocados in a paper bag and leave to ripen at room temperature for several days. Store ripe avocados in the refrigerator for up to several days.

How to Cut: Cut vertically around the pit. Twist the halves apart. The pit will remain in one of the halves. Put that half on the counter and tap a butcher knife into the pit, just enough to stick. Pick up the avocado and twist the knife. The pit should twist out.

For slices, use a dull table knife and slice the avocado while it's still in its skin without cutting the skin. Scrape out each slice as you go along or all at once. For dips, scoop out the flesh with a spoon.

Uses: Use avocado on salads and sandwiches. Make a guacamole dip and use raw vegetables or baked or fat-free chips to dip. Cut in half and stuff with a cold salad. Once cut, avocado turns brown quickly. Add avocados last to a dish or brush with lemon or lime juice.

Of the nearly 20 foods or food groups that have earned the title of Nutrition Superstar, 3 of them are in the fat group. That might come as a surprise, but all these Nutrition Superstars have a lot more to offer nutritionally than just calories from fat.

Herbed Avocado Dressing

Serving Size: 2 Tbsp, Total Servings: 16

Tired of dull-tasting low-fat dressings? Make your own using creamy avocado and rich-tasting buttermilk. Fresh watercress and parsley add a fresh, spring taste. This dressing is good to pour over fresh green salads, or you can use it to dip an assortment of crunchy, raw vegetables.

1 avocado, peeled, pitted, and cubed	**1/4** cup minced parsley
1/2 cup plain nonfat yogurt	**2** scallions, minced
1/2 cup low-fat buttermilk	**1/2** tsp garlic powder
1/4 cup washed, stemmed, and coarsely chopped watercress	**1/4** tsp dill
	Salt and pepper to taste

1 In a blender, mix all ingredients at high speed for 1 minute. Pour into a container and refrigerate until needed. Keeps in refrigerator 2 days.

PREPARATION
15 minutes

Exchanges
1/2 Fat

Calories 28
  Calories from Fat 18
Total Fat . . . . 2 g
  Saturated Fat . . . . .1 g
Cholesterol . . . . 0 mg
Sodium . . . . 17 mg
Carbohydrate . . . . 2 g
  Dietary Fiber . . . . 1 g
  Sugars . . . . 1 g
Protein . . . . 1 g

Flax, oil and seeds
Flax seed, Serving size: 1 Tbsp

Flax is one of the best sources of the polyunsaturated fats called omega-3 fats. It's also a good source of magnesium.

You can use flax oil, or whole or ground flax seeds. Whole seeds are difficult to digest, so you'll get more nutritional value from milled (ground) flax seed. To grind the seeds, simply put them in a coffee grinder.

How to buy: Flax seed can be purchased in bags or in bulk. Available at natural food stores and some grocery stores.

How to store: Keep in the refrigerator. The seeds contains essential oils that will go rancid if stored for a long time at room temperature.

Flax seeds may be used like sesame seeds to add nutrition and crunch to foods. Whirl in a blender or crush slightly with a rolling pin so they're digested more easily.

- Toss flax seed into muffins and quick breads (about 1/4 cup per recipe).
- Toss flax seed into pancakes and waffle batters.
- Top a fresh salad with flax seed.
- Add flax seed to cold or hot cereal.
- Toast flax seeds briefly in a small skillet until aromatic. Top any fresh cooked vegetable with toasted flax seeds.
- Add to meatloaf and casseroles.

Flax seeds can also be used as an egg replacer:

1 Tbsp flax seed plus 3 Tbsp water = 1 egg. Grind the flax seeds in a coffee grinder. A blender or food processor will not work. Transfer the powdered flax seed to a blender and add the water and blend until emulsified. Use as an egg replacer in baking.

Exchanges, Flax Seed
1/2 Fat

Calories 35
    Calories from Fat 20
Total Fat . . . . 2 g
    Saturated Fat . . . . 0 g
Cholesterol . . . . 0 mg
Sodium . . . . 0 mg
Carbohydrate . . . . 3 g
    Dietary Fiber . . . . 2 g
    Sugars . . . . 0 g
Protein . . . . 1 g

Whole-Wheat Flax Loaf

Serving Size: 1 slice, Total Servings: Makes 1 loaf, 12

The addition of flax seed is not unlike having a slice of bread made with other seeds. This is an easy way to incorporate flax seed into your food plan. Try this bread made into French toast.

1 1/4 cups warm water (115 degrees)	**2** tsp dry milk powder
1 Tbsp dry yeast	**2** Tbsp canola oil
1 Tbsp sugar	**4** cups whole wheat flour
2 tsp salt	**1/4** cup flax seed, crushed in blender

1 Dissolve the yeast in the warm water. Add the sugar and let stand for 5 minutes until frothy.

2 Add the salt, milk powder, oil, and 2 cups flour. Mix well.

3 Add the flax seed and remaining flour. Turn dough out onto a lightly-floured surface.

4 Knead the loaf for about 6–10 minutes until elastic and smooth.

5 Shape into a loaf and place in an oiled 9-inch loaf pan. Cover with a tea towel and set in a warm place to rise (radiator, warm spot in the kitchen). Let rise until double in bulk, about 45 minutes.

6 Preheat the oven to 350°F. Bake the loaf for 45 minutes. Remove the loaf from the oven and cool in the pan for 10 minutes. Turn out onto a rack and cool completely before slicing.

PREPARATION
20 minutes, plus 45 minutes rising time

COOK
45 minutes

Exchanges
2 1/2 Starch

Calories 204	
Calories from Fat 35	
Total Fat . . . . 4 g	
Saturated Fat . . . . 0 g	
Cholesterol . . . . 0 mg	
Sodium . . . . 390 mg	
Carbohydrate . . . . 35 g	
Dietary Fiber . . . . 2 g	
Sugars . . . . 2 g	
Protein . . . . 6 g	

Going Nuts!

Nuts are a non-animal source of protein. They're a great source of vitamin E, folic acid, magnesium, and potassium, and they contain some fiber.

Buying and Storing

Buy nuts from a store where you know the merchandise turnover is high. This is your best assurance that the nuts will not be rancid. Buy small quantities.

If you are planning on snacking on nuts, buy them in the shell; it will take a lot more effort to overindulge in them! The shells should not have cracks or holes in them. And nuts, except for peanuts, should not rattle when shaken.

Shelled nuts are sold raw, dry roasted, oil roasted, and salted.

Nuts can be kept in a cool, dry place for several months. They keep best in the refrigerator in a tightly-tied plastic bag or in a jar with a tight-fitting lid. When frozen, nuts will keep for a year or longer.

Uses

We think the best way to incorporate nuts into your food choices is to cook with them. This way you can get their benefits but perhaps will eat less than if you just snack on handfuls.

You can intensify their flavors by toasting them. Put the nuts in a dry, nonstick skillet. Over medium heat, toast the nuts, shaking the pan frequently, until the nuts become golden brown, about 3–5 minutes for most nuts. Store the toasted nuts in the refrigerator for several weeks or put in an airtight package and store in the freezer for 2–3 months.

Sprinkle nuts into salads, soups, stews, main dishes, and baked goods.

Almonds: Almonds are a good source of calcium and monounsaturated fat. Almonds are great tossed into stir-fries, chopped fine and used as a coating for fish, or eaten out of hand.

Brazil nuts: One of the largest nuts, they also pack a few more calories per unit weight. They come in very dark and hard three-sided shells.

Cashews: Cashews are actually toxic because the raw nuts contain prussic acid. They are always processed to rid the nut of its prussic acid, and are sold only shelled because their shells contain prussic acid as well. You can still buy cashews in their raw state, but they will be treated to eliminate the prussic acid. They are great to use in quick-cooking dishes, as prolonged heat will soften them up too much, so put them in at the end. Cashews are high in monounsaturated fat and vitamin E.

Chestnuts: Most people don't lump this old Christmas favorite with other nuts. Chestnuts are mainly carbohydrate and are much lower in fat and calories than the other nuts. They can be enjoyed roasted and eaten from the shell, shelled and used in stuffings, or pureéd and used for soup. Canned chestnuts are also easy to use because the shell has been removed and the chestnut is ready for use. They are available canned.

Coconuts: Coconuts are drupes, not nuts. Coconuts contain mostly artery-clogging saturated fats. Use coconut very sparingly.

Filberts: Filberts and hazelnuts are essentially the same, except hazelnuts are smaller. They are excellent in baking.

Macadamia nuts: These rank among many people's favorites, but I would use them very rarely; their fat and calorie count is very high for a small, 15-piece serving.

Peanuts: Peanuts are actually legumes, relatives of peas and beans, not nuts. Peanuts are great tossed into stir-fries or used in baking. They are a good source of monounsaturated fat.

Pecans: Pecans turn rancid quickly, so use them up fast. They are popular among bakers for pecan pie.

Pine nuts: Also known as pignoli nuts, these nuts are a labor of love. Each nut grows inside a pine cone and is removed by hand, thus making them expensive. Fortunately most recipes will call for only a small amount. They turn rancid easily, so store them in the freezer.

Pistachios: The red dye often found on pistachios has an interesting story. It is used to distinguish them from other nuts in a mixed-nut bowl! Pistachios are a Middle Eastern import but now are grown in California.

Walnuts: We use the most popular form of walnuts, the English or Persian walnut. Most walnuts are now grown in California. They are great for baking. Walnuts have omega-3 fats.

New Waldorf Salad

Serving Size: about 3/4 cup, Total Servings: 4

We call this "new" Waldorf salad because we have lowered the fat content of this famous side salad. We still use all the traditional ingredients, but we use fat-free mayonnaise and fewer nuts. Make a turkey sandwich on whole grain bread and eat this as the sensational side!

2	cups diced apple	**1/2**	cup fat-free mayonnaise
1/2	cup toasted walnuts		Salt and pepper to taste
1	cup sliced celery	**2**	tsp lemon juice
1/4	cup raisins		Red leaf lettuce leaves

1 In a salad bowl, combine the apples, walnuts, celery, and raisins.

2 In a small bowl, mix together the mayonnaise, salt, pepper, and lemon juice.

3 Toss the dressing with the apple-nut mixture.

4 Serve the salad over lettuce leaves.

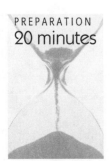

PREPARATION
20 minutes

Exchanges
1 1/2 Fruit
2 Fat

Calories 186
   Calories from Fat 86
Total Fat . . . . .10 g
   Saturated Fat . . . . 0 g
Cholesterol . . . . 0 mg
Sodium . . . . 241 mg
Carbohydrate . . . . 25 g
   Dietary Fiber . . . . 3 g
   Sugars . . . . .16 g
Protein . . . . 3 g

Chinese Chicken with Cashews

Serving Size: about 4 ounces, Total Servings: 4

Making Chicken with Cashews yourself will certainly put the reins on unwanted calories and fat. This one-pot stir-fry needs only the addition of cooked brown rice. By using vegetable spray to stir-fry the vegetables and chicken, you also save the excess fat. A small amount of aromatic sesame oil is used at the end to tie all the flavors together.

2 medium onions, sliced vertically	3 Tbsp lite soy sauce
1 cup broccoli florets	1/3 cup fat-free, reduced-sodium chicken broth
1 lb boneless, skinless chicken breasts, cut into 2-inch cubes	2 tsp rice vinegar
3 green onions, minced	1/2 cup toasted cashews
2 tsp minced ginger	2 tsp sesame oil
3 garlic cloves, minced	

1 Spray a wok or heavy skillet with nonstick cooking spray. Over medium-high heat, add the onions to the pan and sauté for 5 minutes. Remove the onions from the pan.

2 Add more spray and stir-fry the broccoli for 3 minutes. Remove the broccoli from the pan. Add more spray and stir-fry the chicken until it's no longer pink, about 7–8 minutes. Add the green onions, ginger, and garlic and stir-fry for 2 minutes. Add the onions and broccoli back into the pan.

3 Add the soy sauce, broth, and vinegar. Cook for 1 minute.

4 Add the cashews and sesame oil and cook for 1 minute.

PREPARATION
20 minutes

COOK
20 minutes

Exchanges
4 Lean Meat   2 Vegetable
1/2 Fat

Calories 282
   Calories from Fat 119
Total Fat . . . . 13 g
   Saturated Fat . . . . .3 g
Cholesterol . . . . 68 mg
Sodium . . . . 671 mg
Carbohydrate . . . . .12 g
   Dietary Fiber . . . . .2 g
   Sugars . . . . .5 g
Protein . . . . .29 g

Lower-fat Party Foods

Anytime Can Be Party Time!

Even if you eat a low-fat diet, you might feel that dips and snacks have to be high fat. Try these recipes. We're betting you won't notice you've skipped much of the fat.

Sun-dried Tomato Spread

Serving Size: 2 Tbsp, Total Servings: 16

Little bits of earthy sun-dried tomatoes dot this ultra-rich tasting spread. Use to spread on crackers or pita bread.

1	cup fat-free cream cheese
1/2	cup fat-free mayonnaise
3	Tbsp fat-free milk
1/2	cup low-fat sour cream
1/2	cup rehydrated sun-dried tomatoes, sliced
2	tsp minced chives
1	tsp minced thyme
2	tsp minced basil
	Salt and pepper to taste

1 In a food processor, blend all ingredients until smooth but thick. Serve with crackers or raw vegetables of choice.

PREPARATION
10 minutes

Exchanges
1/2 Carbohydrate

Calories 34
   Calories from Fat 6
Total Fat . . . . .1 g
   Saturated Fat . . . . .0 g
Cholesterol . . . . .5 mg
Sodium . . . . .149 mg
Carbohydrate . . . . .4 g
   Dietary Fiber . . . . .0 g
   Sugars . . . . .2 g
Protein . . . . .3 g

Smoky Cheese Dip

Serving Size: 2 Tbsp, Total Servings: 16

You'll need to cook up some low-fat turkey sausage before making this dip. You can omit it if you like—the Worcestershire sauce and liquid smoke are what really gives this dip that smoky taste.

1 cup fat-free cream cheese	1/2 cup cooked crumbled low-fat turkey sausage
1 cup fat-free sour cream	
1/2 cup fat-free mayonnaise	1 tsp Worcestershire sauce
1/2 cup reduced-fat shredded cheddar cheese	1/2 tsp liquid smoke flavoring
	2 cloves garlic, minced

1 In a food processor, combine the cream cheese, sour cream, and mayonnaise. Process until smooth.

2 Fold in by hand the remaining ingredients. Serve with crackers or pita bread.

PREPARATION
10 minutes

Exchanges
1/2 Carbohydrate

Calories 50	
Calories from Fat 8	
Total Fat . . . . 1 g	
Saturated Fat . . . . 1 g	
Cholesterol . . . . 7 mg	
Sodium . . . . 224 mg	
Carbohydrate . . . . 5 g	
Dietary Fiber . . . . 0 g	
Sugars . . . . 2 g	
Protein . . . . 5 g	

Hot Artichoke Dip
Serving Size: 2 Tbsp, Total Servings: 16

Serve this appetizer at your next gathering instead of a cold spread. When blended, artichokes take on a very creamy texture, making this dip thick and rich. You can prepare this recipe up to step 2, cover, and put in the refrigerator up to 24 hours ahead of baking.

2 (15-oz) cans artichoke hearts, drained, reserve 2 Tbsp liquid

2 Tbsp lemon juice

1/3 cup fat-free mayonnaise

2 Tbsp olive oil

1/4 cup Parmesan cheese

1 cup fine dry bread crumbs

1 tsp hot pepper sauce

1 tsp dried oregano

1 tsp dried basil

1 tsp dried thyme

Salt and pepper to taste

1 Preheat oven to 350°F. In a food processor or blender, blend together the artichoke hearts, lemon juice, mayonnaise, olive oil, and Parmesan cheese. Blend for 1 minute until smooth.

2 By hand fold in the remaining ingredients.

3 Pour into a small non-stick casserole dish. Bake for 20–25 minutes until puffed and browned. Serve with crackers or French bread.

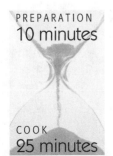
PREPARATION
10 minutes

COOK
25 minutes

Exchanges
1/2 Carbohydrate
1/2 Fat

Calories 62
  Calories from Fat 23
Total Fat . . . . 3 g
  Saturated Fat . . . . 1 g
Cholesterol . . . . 2 mg
Sodium . . . . 214 mg
Carbohydrate . . . . 8 g
  Dietary Fiber . . . . 1 g
  Sugars . . . . 1 g
Protein . . . . 2 g

Hummus

Serving Size: 2 Tbsp, Total Servings: 12

Much less fat than the store or deli versions. Serve with your favorite crackers or whole-wheat pita bread.

1 (15-oz) can chickpeas, drained, reserve 1 Tbsp liquid

3-6 cloves garlic, minced

1 Tbsp sesame tahini

Juice of 1 lemon

2 tsp olive oil

Pinch cayenne pepper

1 Combine all ingredients into a blender until smooth, using the 1 Tbsp chickpea liquid if necessary to make a smooth spread.

PREPARATION
5 minutes

Exchanges
1/2 Carbohydrate

Calories 49
  Calories from Fat 17
Total Fat . . . . 2 g
  Saturated Fat . . . . 0 g
Cholesterol . . . . 0 mg
Sodium . . . . 33 mg
Carbohydrate . . . . 7 g
  Dietary Fiber . . . . 2 g
  Sugars . . . . 1 g
Protein . . . . 2 g

Creamy Spinach Dip

Serving Size: 2 Tbsp, Total Servings: 16

Hollow out a round loaf of unsliced bread. Fill the bread with this dip and watch how fast it goes. Drain the spinach really well so the dip is creamy with no excess water. Use frozen chopped broccoli instead of spinach if you like.

1	(10-oz) package frozen chopped spinach, thawed and drained very well	**2**	Tbsp minced mint
1 1/2	cups low-fat sour cream	**2**	garlic cloves, minced
2	Tbsp red wine vinegar	**1/2**	cup minced water chestnuts
		1/4	tsp cayenne pepper
			Salt and pepper to taste

1 Prepare the spinach and set aside.

2 In a medium bowl, combine the sour cream, vinegar, mint, garlic, water chestnuts, cayenne pepper, salt, and pepper.

3 Add the spinach and mix well. Cover and refrigerate for 1 hour before serving.

PREPARATION
10 minutes

CHILL
1 hour

Exchanges
1/2 Carbohydrate

Calories 33
   Calories from Fat 17
Total Fat . . . . 2 g
   Saturated Fat . . . . 1 g
Cholesterol . . . . 7 mg
Sodium . . . . 27 mg
Carbohydrate . . . . 3 g
   Dietary Fiber . . . . 1 g
   Sugars . . . . 1 g
Protein . . . . 2 g

Potato Skin Bar

Serving Size: 1/2 of a medium potato, Total Servings: 8

Make your own potato skins, then set out an array of toppings and you have the makings of a potato party!

4 medium russet potatoes

4 tsp olive oil

4 Tbsp reduced-fat cheddar cheese

1 Preheat the oven to 350°F. Wash the potatoes and place them directly on the rack. Bake for about 1 hour.

2 Remove the potatoes and cut in half lengthwise. Scoop out the filling, leaving about 1/4 inch of potato. Make mashed potatoes from the filling.

3 Using scissors, cut each potato skin in half again lengthwise. Place all the skins on a baking sheet. Drizzle the olive oil on all the skins.

4 Top each skin with some cheese. Place the skins under a hot broiler for 1–2 minutes until crisp.

Toppings (Set out these toppings—guests can help themselves.)

1/2 cup minced green onions

1/2 cup salsa

1/2 cup low-fat sour cream

1/4 cup cooked crisp turkey bacon

Several dashes of hot sauce

PREPARATION
5 minutes

COOK
1 hour

Exchanges, without toppings
1 Starch

Calories	78
Calories from Fat	25
Total Fat	3 g
Saturated Fat	1 g
Cholesterol	3 mg
Sodium	34 mg
Carbohydrate	11 g
Dietary Fiber	2 g
Sugars	0 g
Protein	2 g

Open-faced Mini Bagel Bar

Serving Size: 1/2 bagel, Total Servings: 4

Have fun with mini bagels. The size of bagels has swelled considerably over the years, giving us more calories and carbohydrates than we really need for a serving. However, getting your bagel fix is just moments away with these inventive little snack sandwiches.

Veggie Sandwich

2 mini bagels

1/4 cup reduced-fat cream cheese (Neufchâtel)

1 tsp Dijon mustard

1 Tbsp minced green onions

Dash hot sauce

16 thin slices cucumber

4 slices tomato

1/4 cup alfalfa sprouts

1 Split the bagels in half.

2 In a small bowl, combine the cream cheese, mustard, green onions, and hot sauce and mix well.

3 Spread the cream cheese mixture evenly on all four bagel halves.

4 Top with slices of cucumber, then tomato. Garnish with sprouts.

PREPARATION
10 minutes (except pizza bagel, 1–2 minutes)

Exchanges, Veggie Sandwich

1/2 Starch   1/2 Fat

Calories 76
  Calories from Fat 30
Total Fat . . . . 3 g
  Saturated Fat . . . . 2 g
Cholesterol . . . . 10 mg
Sodium . . . . 161 mg
Carbohydrate . . . . 8 g
  Dietary Fiber . . . . 1 g
  Sugars . . . . 2 g
Protein . . . . 3 g

Turkey Chutney Sandwich

   2 mini bagels

   1/4 cup reduced-fat cream cheese (Neufchâtel)

   2 Tbsp mango or cranberry chutney

   Dash hot sauce

   1/4 tsp ground ginger

   8 thin slices cucumber

   4 oz sliced turkey

1 Split the bagels in half.

2 In a small bowl, combine the cream cheese, chutney, hot sauce, and ginger. Spread some of the cream cheese mixture over each bagel half.

3 Place 2 slices of cucumber over the cream cheese. Top with a turkey slice.

Tomato Pizza Bagels

   2 mini bagels

   4 Tbsp favorite tomato sauce

   1/2 tsp dried oregano

   4 slices tomato

   4 oz part-skim mozzarella cheese

   1 Tbsp Parmesan cheese

1 Split the bagels in half. Spread some of the tomato sauce over each bagel half. Sprinkle the sauce with oregano. Top with a slice of tomato, cheese, and a sprinkle of Parmesan cheese.

2 Put the bagel halves on a small, nonstick baking sheet.

3 Broil for 1–2 minutes until cheese melts.

Exchanges, Turkey Chutney Sandwich
1 Carbohydrate   1 Lean Meat

Calories	149
Calories from Fat	42
Total Fat	5 g
Saturated Fat	2 g
Cholesterol	32 mg
Sodium	235 mg
Carbohydrate	14 g
Dietary Fiber	0 g
Sugars	5 g
Protein	11 g

Exchanges, Tomato Pizza Bagels
1/2 Starch   1 Medium-fat Meat

Calories	124
Calories from Fat	49
Total Fat	5 g
Saturated Fat	3 g
Cholesterol	18 mg
Sodium	297 mg
Carbohydrate	10 g
Dietary Fiber	1 g
Sugars	2 g
Protein	9 g

Low-fat Buffalo Wings

Serving Size: 2 oz chicken, Total Servings: 4

At colleges in upstate New York, chicken wings were almost as big a part of the college experience as getting a degree. Traditional buffalo wings have so much fat, we don't care to even let you know! Here you can significantly lower the fat content. Don't forget the blue cheese dressing; it makes these buffalo wings authentic!

1 1/2	Tbsp hot sauce	**1/4**	tsp paprika
	Pinch cayenne	**1/2**	lb chicken tenders

Dressing

1/2 cup reduced-fat blue cheese dressing

1/4 cup low-fat mayonnaise

3 Tbsp crumbled blue cheese

Celery sticks

1 Preheat the oven to 375°F. In a shallow bowl, combine the hot sauce, cayenne, and paprika. Roll the chicken tenders in the mixture.

2 Place the chicken tenders on a small nonstick baking sheet. Bake, uncovered, for 15 minutes until chicken is tender.

3 Combine the dressing ingredients. Serve the dressing with the chicken and celery sticks.

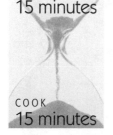

PREPARATION
15 minutes

COOK
15 minutes

Exchanges
1/2 Carbohydrate
2 Medium-fat Meat

Calories 192
   Calories from Fat 104
Total Fat . . . . .12 g
   Saturated Fat . . . . .3 g
Cholesterol . . . . 42 mg
Sodium . . . . 572 mg
Carbohydrate . . . . 7 g
   Dietary Fiber . . . . 0 g
   Sugars . . . . 4 g
Protein . . . . 14 g

	Exchange/ Serving	Calories	Total Fat (g)	Sat. Fat (g)	Mono. Fat (g)	Poly Fat (g)	Cholesterol (mg)
Monounsaturated Fats							
Almonds, dry roasted	6 whole	47	4	0.5	2.5	1	0
Avocado	1/8	40	4	0.5	2.5	0.5	0
Cashews, salted	6 whole	52	4	1	2.5	0.5	0
Mixed nuts (<50% peanuts)	6 nuts	37	3.5	0.5	2	1	0
Oils							
Canola	1 tsp	41	4.5	0.5	3	1.5	0
Olive	1 tsp	40	4.5	0.5	3.5	0.5	0
Peanut	1 tsp	40	4.5	1	2	1.5	0
Olives, green, stuffed, large (sodium)	10	50	4	0.5	3	0.5	0
Olives, ripe, large	8	40	3.5	0.5	3	0.5	0
Peanuts, dry roasted	10 nuts	44	4.5	0.5	2	1.5	0
Peanut butter, smooth	2 tsp	63	5.5	1	2.5	1.5	0
Pecans	4 halves	46	4.5	0.5	3	1	0
Sesame seeds	1 Tbsp	52	4.5	0.5	1.5	2	0
Tahini paste	2 tsp	59	5.5	1	2	2.5	0
Polyunsaturated Fats							
Margarine, stick, >80% veg. oil	1 tsp	34	4	0.5	1.5	1	0
Margarine, tub, >75% veg. oil	1 tsp	30	3.5	0.5	0.5	1.5	0
Margarine, squeeze, >70% veg. oil	1 tsp	30	3.5	0.5	1	1.5	0
Margarine, lower-fat, 30-50% veg. oil	1 Tbsp	50	6	1	1.5	1.5	0
Margarine, reduced-calorie	1 Tbsp	50	5.5	1	3	2	0
Mayonnaise	1 tsp	33	3.5	0.5	1	2	3
Mayonnaise, light/reduced-fat	1 Tbsp	40	3	0.5	1.5	2.5	6
Miracle Whip salad dressing, regular	2 tsp	39	3.5	0.5	1	2	3
Miracle Whip, reduced-calorie	1 Tbsp	45	4	1	1	2	5

(continued)

Fats

	Exchange/ Serving	Calories	Total Fat (g)	Sat. Fat (g)	Mono. Fat (g)	Poly Fat (g)	Cholesterol (mg)
Polyunsaturated Fats (cont'd)							
Oils							
Corn	1 tsp	44	5	0.5	1	3	0
Safflower	1 tsp	44	5	0.5	0.5	3.5	0
Soybean	1 tsp	44	5	0.5	1	3	0
Pumpkin seeds, roasted	1 Tbsp	70	5.5	1	2	2.5	0
Sunflower seeds, dry roasted	1 Tbsp	47	4	0.5	1	2.5	0
Walnuts, English	4 halves	51	5	0.5	1	3	0
Saturated Fats							
Bacon, fried, drained	1 slice	35	3	1	1.5	0.5	5
Bacon grease	1 tsp	36	4	1.5	2	0.5	4
Butter, stick	1 tsp	36	4	2.5	1	0	11
Chitterlings, boiled	2 Tbsp	42	4	1.5	1.5	1	20
Coconut, shredded, dried, sweetened	2 Tbsp	52	3.5	3	0	0	0
Cream, half-and-half	2 Tbsp	39	3.5	2	1	0	11
Cream cheese, regular	1 Tbsp	49	5	3	1.5	0	15
Cream cheese, reduced-fat	2 Tbsp	60	5	3	1.5	0	15
Lard	1 tsp	36	4	1.5	1.5	0.5	4
Salt pork, raw, cured	1/4 oz	52	5.5	2	2.5	0.5	6
Shortening	1 tsp	35	4	1	2	1	0
Sour cream, regular	2 Tbsp	52	5	3	1.5	0	10
Sour cream, reduced-fat	3 Tbsp	45	3.5	2.5	1	0	15

(sodium) = 400 mg or more of sodium per exchange.

Sugars, Sweets, and Sweeteners

RECIPES

Carob Brownies ———————————— 268

Old-Fashioned Spiced Banana Bread———— 269

Just Peachy Crisp———————————— 270

OK TO EAT?

When people hear "diabetes," what's the first bit of nutrition advice they expect to hear? "Avoid sugars and sweets," of course.

The good news is that this nutrition advice is out-of-date. The bad news is it will be a long time before this dogma dies.

Until then, turn to the experts for answers. And when you're savoring a sweet dessert and a well-meaning friend or relative leans over to say, "Shouldn't you stay away from sweets?" do everyone else with diabetes a favor and bring their knowledge into the 21st century.

WHAT ARE SUGARS AND SWEETS?

"Sugars" are the sweeteners you find in your pantry (granulated sugar, brown sugar, honey, maple syrup), and the sweeteners used in commercial food products (high-fructose corn syrup, corn sweeteners, and dextrose).

"Sugary foods" are regular soda, gum drops, jelly, and fruit drinks.

"Sweets" are cake, cookies, pies, and the like. Sweets usually contain fat. And it's the fat that sends the calories in sweets skyrocketing, not the sugars.

WHAT DOES THE AMERICAN DIABETES ASSOCIATION SAY?

Research studies conducted from the mid-1970s to the present have shown that gram for gram, sugars don't raise blood glucose any more quickly than do other sources of carbohydrate.

With this overwhelming research in mind, the current American Diabetes Association nutrition recommendations state that it is **the total amount of carbohydrate you eat that most affects blood glucose**, not the type or source of carbohydrate. A phrase that has been popularized is "carbohydrate equals carbohydrate equals carbohydrate."

Is this advice designed to promote a sugar and sweets free-for-all? Certainly not! People with diabetes are, like all Americans, encouraged to eat sugars and sweets only in moderation. That's because foods with lots of sugars don't offer much in the way of nutrition, they often have a lot of fat, and some of it is unhealthy fat at that.

If you simply are not a sweets eater, then continue to stay away from them. If, on the other hand, you can't live without sweets, feel comfortable enjoying them once in a while using these guidelines:

- Substitute sugary foods or sweets for other carbohydrates in your meal plan. In other words, if you choose to eat a sweet, lighten up on other carbohydrates in the meal—have less bread, potato, or fruit.

- Counterbalance the calories from sweets by burning more calories with extra activity.

NUTRITION NUMBERS FOR AMERICA'S 10 FAVORITE DESSERTS

Food	Serving Size	Calories	Carbohydrate (g)	Fat (g)
Apple pie a la mode	1 slice (1/8 pie), plus 1/2 cup ice cream	376	45	21
Pecan pie	1 slice	503	64	27
Ice cream sundae	Medium	459	57	24
Chocolate chip cookie	1 large	235	35	9
Chocolate layer cake with frosting	1 slice	308	37	16
Donut, glazed	1	254	29	14
Peach cobbler	3x3 inch piece	210	36	6
Cheesecake	1 slice	257	20	18
Brownies with walnuts	2" square	168	18	11
Pound cake	1 slice	230	25	13

You'll want to eat sweets while still reaching your nutrition and diabetes goals, so consider the following:

- Limit sugary and sweet foods until you get your blood glucose under control.

- If a goal for you is to lose some weight, then you'll need to keep sweets to a once-in-a-while frequency. Too many sweets means too many calories.

- If your total cholesterol, LDL, HDL, and triglycerides are not where you want them, keep sweets to a minimum because sweets contain fats. Get your blood lipids under control before you up the number of sweets.

Tips to Limit Sweets

- Choose just a few favorite desserts and decide how often you will eat them.

- Satisfy your sweet tooth with a small portion of your favorite sweet.

- If you have a hard time limiting portions or frequency, it's best to keep large portions of sweets out of the house. Buy a small quantity at a time, or have dessert only at restaurants.

- Split a dessert in a restaurant. Ask for several forks or spoons.

- Take advantage of smaller portions—kiddie, small, or regular—at ice cream shops or in the supermarket.

- Check your blood glucose from time to time about one to two hours after you eat a sweet to see how high it makes your blood glucose rise.

- Try to satisfy your sweet tooth without sugar (or fat!) with: sugar-free popsicles or fudgsicles, sugar-free hot cocoa, sugar-free gelatin, low- or no-sugar jelly, sugar-free powdered drink mixes.

Tips to Limit Sugars

Sugars can sometimes creep in without you realizing it. They contribute calories and carbohydrate which makes blood glucose rise.

- Instead of regular soda, drink diet soda, or better yet, water.

- Instead of fruit drink, drink 100% fruit juice, or better yet, eat pieces of fruit.

- Skip the canned fruit packed in heavy syrup; get fruit packed in its own juice or light syrup.

- When you order or buy iced tea make sure it is unsweetened.

- When you buy fruit drinks or flavored seltzers, read the nutrition label and make sure the calories, carbohydrate, and sugars are near zero.

- Use the low-calorie sweetener of your choosing instead of sugar.

- Use low- or no-sugar jelly or jam instead of regular.

SUGAR-FREE SWEETENERS

You're cruising the supermarket aisles. The words "sugar-free" and "no-added-sugar" in big, bold, red print beg you to put your hands around the package and drop it into your supermarket cart. Before you fill your cupboard, refrigerator, and freezer with sugar-free and no-added-sugar foods you need to know the facts.

Sugar Alcohols

Some of the foods you see have sugar alcohols. Sugar alcohols are neither sugars nor alcohol. Sugar alcohols are carbohydrates that have a lower calorie count than other carbohydrates. Sugar alcohols provide on average 2 calories per gram, whereas other carbohydrates (including sugar) are 4 calories per gram.

Sugar alcohols are used by food manufacturers to replace either sugars or fat to create foods that are lower in calories, sugar, and/or fat. Oftentimes they are used to replace the bulk or volume that sugar gives products.

Another name for this category of sweeteners is polyols. The names of polyols are easily recognized in the ingredient list on products because most of the time they end in "ol." Lactitol, mannitol, sorbitol, and xylitol are a few. Isomalt and hydrogenated starch hydrolysates are two polyols that don't end in "ol." Polyols

Q *Is honey better than sugar?*

A *Honey is a source of concentrated carbohydrates and raises blood glucose as much and as quickly as other forms of sugars. Honey offers no advantages over other sources of sugars.*

Q *Is fructose a good sweetener for people with diabetes?*

A *Fructose, which can be purchased in the supermarket as a sweetener to use on foods or to use in cooking, may not raise blood glucose as quickly or as much as other sugars. However, research has shown that large amounts of fructose can raise total cholesterol and LDL cholesterol. The American Diabetes Association concludes that all in all, fructose has no advantage as a sweetener to people with diabetes.*

are most commonly used in candies, cookies, chewing gum, drinks, puddings, and sugar-free cough drops and breath mints.

Up Sides and Down Sides

Polyols provide fewer calories per gram than other carbohydrates because they are not completely absorbed. This factor leads to a down side: They can cause gas, bloating, and diarrhea if eaten in excess or if your stomach is not used to them. Some people are simply sensitive to polyols.

In theory, polyols won't raise blood glucose levels quite as much as other carbohydrates, but in reality, over the course of a day, they don't offer people with diabetes much of an advantage.

One more plus: Polyols don't promote tooth decay. Two more minuses: Foods with polyols can be more expensive than the regularly sweetened food and not as tasty.

On the Food Label

According to the FDA food labeling regulations, sugar-free means less than 0.5 grams of sugars per serving. Sugars, by definition, do not include sugar alcohols. Products that use sugar alcohols to sweeten the food, rather than sugars, can be labeled sugar-free or no-added-sugar.

On the Nutrition Facts, polyols are counted as part of the Total Carbohydrate. If a manufacturer makes a nutrition claim that the food is sugar-free or has no added sugar, then they must put the grams of sugar alcohols on the Nutrition Facts as a subcategory of Total Carbohydrate.

Fitting In Foods with Polyols

If you choose to use foods with polyols, you need to count them into your meal plan. Use these guidelines to do so.

If the Total Carbohydrate in the food comes from sugar alcohols and there are less than 10 g in a serving:	• Count the food as a free food. • Remember a "free food" is defined as up to 20 calories and up to 5 grams of carbohydrate per serving. Limit "free foods" to 3 or fewer servings per day or the calories and carbohydrate will add up and keep you from meeting your goals.
If the Total Carbohydrate in the food comes from sugar alcohols and the grams of polyols are more than 10:	• Subtract one-half of the grams of sugar alcohols from the Total Carbohydrate. Use the remaining grams of carbohydrate and figure that into your meal plan.

If there are several sources of carbohydrate that includes some from sugar alcohols:

- Subtract one-half of the grams of sugar alcohols from the Total Carbohydrate and count the remaining grams of carbohydrate into your meal plan.

Remember:

- Polyols contain fewer calories, but foods with polyols are not calorie- or carbohydrate-free.

- Don't use foods with polyols to treat low blood glucose (hypoglycemia). These foods will not raise blood glucose quickly enough.

LOW- TO NO-CALORIE SWEETENERS

You may also see the sugar-free and no-added-sugar nutrition claim on products that use low-calorie sweeteners, also called nonnutritive sweeteners, no-calorie sweeteners, or sugar substitutes. They have next-to-no carbohydrate, sugar, or calories. They don't raise blood glucose levels.

Four low-calorie sweeteners are now available in the United States. These sweeteners, on the market after going through the FDA's rigorous food additive approval process, are safe for all people with diabetes, with two exceptions: Women who are pregnant or breastfeeding should not use saccharin, and people with phenylketonuria (PKU) should not use aspartame.

Acesulfame potassium, or ace-k for short

Some people pick up a bitter aftertaste when they eat or drink products with ace-k. To reduce this, some manufacturers use ace-k in combination with another low-calorie sweetener.

Aspartame

Aspartame has a clean sweet taste. A familiar name for aspartame is the brand name NutraSweet. Since 1994, when the patent expired, other companies have been able to manufacture aspartame. It is used to sweeten many foods and beverages.

Saccharin

Saccharin has been used as a non-caloric sweetener in foods and beverages for nearly 100 years. Interestingly, it was used during the sugar shortages of the two world wars, particularly in Europe. Through the 1970s, saccharin was the only low-calorie sweetener available in the United States. A drawback of saccharin is the bitter aftertaste it leaves for some people.

There was an attempt to ban the use of saccharin in the 1970s because of the finding of bladder tumors in rats fed high doses of saccharin. Many years of research on saccharin shows that it is safe to be consumed by humans. Recently, saccharin was taken off the list of carcinogens. There will no longer be a warning label on products with saccharin.

Sucralose

Sucralose (brand name Splenda) was approved by the FDA in 1998. It is the sweetest low-calorie sweetener approved to date at about 600 times the sweetness of sugar. Splenda can substitute for sugar in cooking and baking. It is also used as a sweetening ingredient in many food and beverages.

On the Horizon

Three more non-nutritive sweeteners may come on the market:

- Alitame is a protein-based sweetener. Sufficient research on its safety was completed to file a food additive petition at FDA in 1986.

- Cyclamate was discovered in 1937. It was banned in the United States in 1970 because it was linked to cancer in rats. Upon further research, that doesn't appear to be true. Currently a petition is at the FDA to reapprove cyclamate in the United States. It is currently available in Canada, where, interestingly, saccharin is banned.

- Neotame may offer better sweetness stability than aspartame in many foods and beverages. A food additive petition was filed with FDA in 1997 to approve the use of neotame as a tabletop sweetener and in 1998 to approve the use of neotame as a general purpose sweetener.

Blends: The Future of Low-Calorie Sweeteners

A wide variety of low-calorie sweeteners allows manufacturers to use the sweetener or a blend of two or more sweeteners to create products with improved taste, increased stability on the supermarket shelf, and lower manufacturing costs. You probably don't realize it, but fountain diet soda has been a blend of aspartame and saccharin for many years. And Pepsi introduced Pepsi One in 1998, which uses a blend of ace-k and aspartame. More blends of low-calorie sweeteners will be used in the future.

Fitting In Low-Calorie Sweeteners

When you try to fit products sweetened with low-calorie sweeteners into your meal plan, divide them into three categories as follows:

- The tabletop low-calorie sweeteners usually have about 2 calories for the equivalent of the sweetness of 2 teaspoons of sugar. And the calories are not from the low-calorie sweetener, but from the dextrose or maltodextrin that is used to give bulk or volume to the product. These are negligible calories and are considered free unless huge amounts are consumed. They will not likely contribute to raising blood glucose levels either.

- Foods with low-calorie sweeteners may contain next-to-no calories. Examples are diet soda, diet gelatin, chewing gum, fruit drinks, and powdered drink mix. As long as the Nutrition Facts tell you that a serving has fewer than 20 calories and less than 5 grams of carbohydrate per serving, consider it a free food.

- Some foods sweetened with low-calorie sweeteners contain ingredients other than the sweetener that may contribute carbohydrate, other nutrients, and calories. Examples are hot cocoa mix, fruited yogurt, maple syrup, baked goods, frozen desserts, canned fruit, and fruit drink juice combinations. To fit these foods into your meal plan, read the Nutrition Facts to determine the nutrients in a serving.

Carob Brownies

Serving Size: 1 brownie, Total Servings: 12 brownies

Perfect to make on a rainy day. So easy, we don't know who will make them more—you or your kids!

1/2 cup unsweetened applesauce	**1/3** cup carob powder or cocoa
1/2 cup honey	**2/3** cup unbleached flour
1 egg	**2** tsp baking powder
1 egg white	**1/2** cup chopped walnuts (optional)
1 tsp vanilla	

1 Preheat the oven to 325°F. In a large bowl beat together the applesauce, honey, egg, egg white, and vanilla.

2 In a small bowl, combine the carob, flour, and baking powder. Add to the applesauce mixture. Stir in the nuts. Pour the mixture into an oiled 8 × 8-inch baking pan. Bake for 20–25 minutes. Remove from the oven and cool completely. Cut into squares.

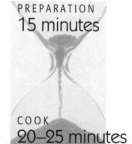

PREPARATION
15 minutes

COOK
20–25 minutes

Exchanges
1 Carbohydrate

Calories 86
  Calories from Fat 7
Total Fat . . . . .1 g
  Saturated Fat . . . . .0 g
Cholesterol . . . . 18 mg
Sodium . . . . .71 mg
Carbohydrate . . . . 20 g
  Dietary Fiber . . . . .1 g
  Sugars . . . . 13 g
Protein . . . . .2 g

Old-fashioned Spiced Banana Bread

Serving Size: 1 (1-inch) slice, Total Servings: 1 (9-inch) loaf

1 1/4 cups all-purpose flour	1/4 tsp salt
1/2 cup whole-wheat flour	1 egg, beaten
1/2 cup sugar	2 bananas, mashed
2 tsp baking powder	3/4 cup unsweetened applesauce
2 tsp cinnamon	2 Tbsp canola oil
1 tsp allspice	1/3 cup fat-free milk
1/2 tsp ginger	

1 Preheat the oven to 350°F. In a large bowl, combine the all-purpose flour, whole-wheat flour, sugar, baking powder, cinnamon, allspice, ginger, and salt.

2 In a medium bowl, combine the eggs, bananas, oil, and milk. Add the banana mixture slowly to the flour mixture and mix until just combined. Don't overbeat.

3 Spray a 9 × 5 × 3-inch loaf pan with nonstick spray. Dust the pan lightly with flour. Pour the batter into the prepared pan.

4 Bake the banana bread for 45–50 minutes until a knife inserted in the center comes out clean. Let the bread cool in the pan for 15 minutes, then turn the loaf out onto a rack and cool completely.

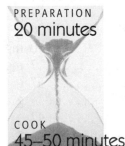

PREPARATION
20 minutes

COOK
45–50 minutes

Exchanges
2 Carbohydrate
1 1/2 Fat

Calories 214
 Calories from Fat 70
Total Fat . . . . 8 g
 Saturated Fat . . . . 0 g
Cholesterol . . . . 47 mg
Sodium . . . . 165 mg
Carbohydrate . . . . 33 g
 Dietary Fiber . . . . 2 g
 Sugars . . . . 16 g
Protein . . . . 4 g

Just Peachy Crisp

Serving Size: 1/4 of crisp, Total Servings: 4

4 medium peaches, unpeeled and sliced thin

1/2 cup fresh blueberries

2 tsp lemon juice

1 cup water

1/3 cup sugar

1 tsp cinnamon

1 1/2 Tbsp cornstarch or arrowroot

Oat Crumb Topping

2 Tbsp flour

1/3 cup rolled oats

1/4 cup brown sugar

2 tsp cinnamon

3 Tbsp canola oil

1 Preheat the oven to 350°F. Grease a casserole dish with a little oil.

2 In a saucepot over medium heat, combine together the peaches, blueberries, lemon juice, water, sugar, cinnamon, and cornstarch.

3 Cook over medium heat until mixture thickens, about 5–8 minutes. Pour the hot fruit into a casserole dish.

4 In a small bowl, mix together the flour, oats, sugar, and cinnamon for the crumb topping. Add the oil and mix well with a fork. Sprinkle the topping over the peaches and bake for 10–15 minutes until peaches are bubbly and crisp topping is lightly browned.

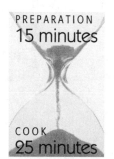

PREPARATION
15 minutes

COOK
25 minutes

Exchanges
3 1/2 Carbohydrate
2 Fat

Calories 327
   Calories from Fat 101
Total Fat . . . . 11 g
   Saturated Fat . . . . 0 g
Cholesterol . . . . 0 mg
Sodium . . . . 7 mg
Carbohydrate . . . . 57 g
   Dietary Fiber . . . . 4 g
   Sugars . . . . 42 g
Protein . . . . 3 g

	Serving	Calories	Carbohydrate (g)	Total Fat (g)	Sat. Fat (g)	Cholesterol (mg)	Exchanges
Angel food cake	1/12 cake	142	32	0	0	0	2 Carbohydrates
Brownie, unfrosted	2" sq	115	18	4.5	1	5	1 Carbohydrate, 1 Fat
Cake, unfrosted	2" sq	97	17	3	0.5	18	1 Carbohydrate, 1 Fat
Cake, frosted	2" sq	175	29	6.5	1.5	18	2 Carbohydrates, 1 Fat
Cupcake, frosted, small	1	172	28	6	1.5	1	2 Carbohydrates, 1 Fat
Donut, plain cake	1	198	23	11	2	18	1 1/2 Carbohydrate, 2 Fats
Donut, glazed (3 3/4" dia)	2 oz	245	27	14	3.5	4	2 Carbohydrates, 2 Fats
Fruit spreads, 100% fruit	1 Tbsp	43	11	0	0	0	1 Carbohydrate
Gelatin, reg. (Jello)	1/2 cup	80	19	0	0	0	1 Carbohydrate
Gingersnaps	3	87	16	2	0.5	0	1 Carbohydrate
Granola bar	1	133	18	5.5	0.7	0	1 Carbohydrate, 1 Fat
Granola bar, fat-free	1	140	35	0	0	0	2 Carbohydrates
Honey	1 Tbsp	64	17	0	0	0	1 Carbohydrate
Ice cream, light	1/2 cup	100	14	4	2.5	25	1 Carbohydrate, 1 Fat
Ice cream, fat-free, no sugar added	1/2 cup	90	20	0	0	0	1 Carbohydrate
Jam or preserves, regular	1 Tbsp	48	13	0	0	0	1 Carbohydrate
Jelly, regular	1 Tbsp	52	14	0	0	0	1 Carbohydrate
Pie, fruit, 2 crusts	1/6 pie	290	43	13	2.5	0	3 Carbohydrates, 2 Fats
Pie, pumpkin or custard	1/8 pie	168	19	8.5	1	21	1 Carbohydrate, 2 Fats
Pudding, regular, low-fat milk	1/2 cup	144	26	2.5	1.5	9	2 Carbohydrates
Pudding, sugar-free, low-fat milk	1/2 cup	90	13	2	1.5	9	1 Carbohydrate

(continued)

Sweets

	Serving	Calories	Carbohydrate (g)	Total Fat (g)	Sat. Fat (g)	Cholesterol (mg)	Exchanges
Sherbet	1/2 cup	132	29	2	1	5	2 Carbohydrates
Sorbet	1/2 cup	130	31	0	0	0	2 Carbohydrates
Sweet roll or Danish	1 (2 1/2 oz)	263	36	11	3	47	2 1/2 Carbohydrates, 2 Fats
Syrup, maple, regular	1 Tbsp	52	13	0	0	0	1 Carbohydrate
Syrup, pancake, light	2 Tbsp	49	13	0	0	0	1 Carbohydrate
Syrup, pancake, regular	1 Tbsp	57	15	0	0	0	1 Carbohydrate
Vanilla wafers	5	88	15	3	0.5	12	1 Carbohydrate, 1 Fat
Yogurt, frozen, fat-free	1/3 cup	60	12	0	0	0	1 Carbohydrate
Yogurt, frozen, fat-free, no sugar added	1/2 cup	90	18	0	0	0	1 Carbohydrate
Yogurt, low-fat, with fruit	1 cup	253	47	3	0.5	10	3 Carbohydrates, 0–1 Fat

FOCUS ON Alcohol

Alcohol is at the tip of the pyramid.
The message is: Use sparingly, if at all.

The American Diabetes Association's position is that the same precautions that apply to the general public also apply to people with diabetes. Dietary Guidelines for Americans recommends that men drink no more than two drinks a day and women drink no more than one drink per day.

One alcoholic beverage is:

- 12 oz beer

- 5 oz wine

- 1 1/2 oz distilled spirits (whiskey, bourbon, gin, etc.).

Of course, abstaining from alcohol is advised for women who are pregnant. Reducing or abstaining from alcohol is also suggested for people with diabetes who have diabetic neuropathy (nerve damage) or abnormal blood fats, especially elevated triglycerides. If you do drink, learn how alcohol may affect your blood glucose levels, learn how to work alcoholic drinks into your meal plan, and drink only in moderation.

Effect on Blood Glucose

Alcohol is not broken down into glucose. In addition, alcohol stops the liver from producing glucose.

Therefore, if you use insulin or a diabetes medication that can cause blood glucose to get too low (hypoglycemia) and you drink alcohol, your blood glucose level may drop too low. This can occur even 8 to 12 hours after you drink. Medications that can cause hypoglycemia are: insulin, sulfonylureas, repaglinide (Prandin), Glucovance, and nateglinide (Starlix).

Don't be fooled! Your blood glucose may go up shortly after drinking if you have a drink that contains carbohydrate, such as beer or a cocktail made with juice. But then hours later, the alcohol may make your blood glucose drop too low.

To be safe:

- Don't drink when your blood glucose is too low.

- Don't drink when your stomach is empty.

If you do drink and you use diabetes medications that can cause hypoglycemia:

- Check your blood glucose level before you drink. This helps you decide if you should drink and to know whether you need to eat something before you drink.

- Be aware of when your medications are at their peak action, that is, having the most action of lowering blood glucose. You are more susceptible to hypoglycemia from alcohol during this time.

- Drink alcohol with your usual meal or snack.

- Don't substitute alcohol for carbohydrate.

- Check your blood glucose level more frequently while you're drinking and for a number of hours after you drink.

- Wear medical I.D. The symptoms of too much alcohol and low blood glucose can be similar. You want people to give you the right treatment if your blood glucose gets too low.

- Check your blood glucose level before you go to sleep. If it's low, eat a snack to prevent low blood glucose during the night. Some people find they need to eat 15 grams of carbohydrate for every drink they had during the evening.

If Weight Gain Is a Concern

Alcohol offers little in the way of nutrition other than calories, and those add up quickly. Look at the calories from alcohol consumed during this restaurant meal:

Before-dinner cocktail: 1 rum-and-diet cola (1 1/2 oz rum), 96 calories

During dinner: 2 glasses white wine (5 oz), 200 calories

After-dinner: brandy (1 1/2 oz), 96 calories

Total: about 400 calories

So alcohol can pack on the pounds. If you are trying to lose or not gain weight, alcohol is best substituted for fat in the meal plan, with one drink counting as 2 fat exchanges. And avoid the calories that often go along with alcohol:

- Use non-caloric mixers—club soda, diet tonic water, water, coffee, or diet soda.

- Keep a no-calorie beverage by your side to quench your thirst.

- Avoid sugar-loaded drinks: those made with syrups, liqueurs, cordials, and regular soda; pre-mixed drinks such as wine coolers; drinks made with sugar-loaded mixes such as daiquiris and whiskey sours.

NUTRITION PROFILE FOR ALCOHOLIC BEVERAGES

Category	Amount	Calories	Carbohydrate (g)	Exchange/ Serving
Beer, regular	12 oz	140	13	1 Carbohydrate, 2 Fats
Beer, light	12 oz	99	5	2 Fats
Wine, red	5 oz	106	3	2 Fats
Wine, white	5 oz	100	1	2 Fats
Wine, rose	5 oz	105	2	2 Fats
Liquor, whiskey, bourbon, scotch, gin, vodka, rum	1 1/2 oz	96	0	2 Fats
Liqueur/cordial	1 1/2 oz	159	20	1 Carbohydrate, 2 Fats
Brandy	1 1/2 oz	96	0	2 Fats
Wine cooler, premixed	12 oz	169	20	1 Carbohydrate, 2 Fats
Mixed drink, screwdriver	6 oz	150	16	1 Carbohydrate, 2 Fats

Two Weeks of Menus

To help you see how to plan meals and daily menus that meet your nutrition needs, we've created 14 days of sample menus for three different calorie ranges. The menus use many of the recipes in this book, so you'll see how to fit in Nutty Blueberry Pancakes, Cheese Polenta, and Healthy Coleslaw. Let these meal plans and menus paint you a picture of what healthy meals look like.

CALORIES

To determine the number of calories you need to eat, check the chart on page 294. Also work with a dietitian or other health care provider to determine your calorie needs. In these menus, the calories are distributed into about 50% carbohydrate, 20% protein, and 30% fat. Your daily food choices for your calorie range are:

■ 1,200–1,400 Calorie Range
174 g carbohydrate, 68 g protein, 35 g fat

6 Starch, 3 Vegetable, 3 Fruit, 2 Milk, 4 Meat, 3 Fat

■ 1,600–1,800 Calorie Range
209 g carbohydrate, 80 g protein, 60 g fat

7 Starch, 4 Vegetable, 4 Fruit, 2 Milk, 5 Meat, 7 Fat

■ 2,000–2,200 Calorie Range
254 g carbohydrate, 96 g protein, 75 g fat

10 Starch, 4 Vegetable, 4 Fruit, 2 Milk, 6 Meat, 9 Fat

CARBOHYDRATE

Many people with diabetes find it easier to reach their blood glucose goals when they keep their carbohydrate intake consistent, so the meal plans here have consistent carbohydrate content. The menus show the huge variety you can have in meals while keeping carbohydrate content consistent.

The way we have divided the servings/exchanges and amount of carbohydrate at each meal simply represents one option. Many others exist.

For those of you who use or want to use carbohydrate counting as your approach to diabetes meal planning, we've provided both the grams of carbohydrate and carbohydrate choices for each meal. You'll note that these don't add up the same. When people count grams of carbohydrate, they count all the grams of carbohydrate in a meal. When people count carbohydrate choices, they count 1 serving/1 exchange of starch, fruit, or milk as 1 carbohydrate choice. They don't count the carbohydrate from vegetables unless 3 servings of vegetables are eaten in a meal, which adds up to 1 carbohydrate choice.

Some of the recipes show you that 1 serving equals 1 carbohydrate rather than specifically a starch or a fruit. That's because the recipe contains a mixture of carbohydrate-containing foods, perhaps some vegetable, grain, and fruit. In the menus we've counted these recipes more with the total grams of carbohydrate in mind while still maintaining the healthiness of the meal.

FAT

The fat content of these meals is *not* consistent—because it doesn't need to be. Fat has little effect on blood glucose. You can be flexible with how you divide fat throughout the day and how much you use on different days, within limits. The number of fat grams and servings/exchanges are provided as a total for the day.

MEAT

The meat servings/exchanges in these meals were calculated based on medium-fat meats, which contain 75 calories, 7 grams of protein, and 5 grams of fat. They are all cooked quantities. If you choose lower-fat or higher-fat meats, you will eat fewer or more calories, respectively. In some of the menus, one meat serving/exchange from lunch or dinner is used for breakfast. The total number of servings/exchanges for the day still add up correctly.

SNACKS

These menu plans don't contain snacks. If you eat snacks, either because you want to or because your diabetes plan calls for snacks, then use one or two of the servings from the meals as snack servings. For example, a piece of fruit and/or starch serving, or a starch and/or milk serving.

MILK

Two servings/exchanges of milk per day are generally used in each of these meal and menu plans. This amount of milk is recommended for adequate calcium intake. If you don't drink or tolerate milk, you can swap one serving of milk for about 1 starch and 1/2 very lean meat serving/exchange. We've done that on some of the menus where noted.

HEALTHY EATING

The foods selected for these menus are based on the nutrition goals recommended throughout this book, such as choose more high-fiber foods and choose foods to keep your saturated fat intake under 10%.

Two Weeks of Menus for 1,200–1,400 Calorie Range

Breakfast: 57 grams carbohydrate/4 Carbohydrate Choices/2 Starch, 1 Fruit, 1 Milk

Lunch: 50 grams carbohydrate/3 Carbohydrate Choices/2 Starch, 1 Vegetable, 1 Fruit, 2 Meat

Dinner: 67 grams carbohydrate/4 Carbohydrate Choices/2 Starch, 2 Vegetable, 1 Fruit, 1 Milk, 2 Meat

	Day 1	Day 2	Day 3

Breakfast	1 cup bran flakes
	2 Tbsp raisins
	1 cup fat-free milk
		3/4 cup/1 serving
		  Strawberry Almond
		  Shake (p. 134)
		1 fat-free granola bar
		1 small banana
			1/2 grapefruit
			1/2 cup grits
			2 slices whole-wheat
			  toast with 1 fried egg
			  with 1 tsp margarine
			(Egg and 1 starch substi-
			  tutes for 1 milk.)

Lunch	1 cup green salad with
	2 Tbsp reduced-fat salad
	  dressing
	1 Beef Stroganoff frozen
	  entree
	1/2 pear (4 oz)
		1 cup sliced cucumbers
		1 cup Quinoa Salad
		  (p. 35)
		1/2 cup low-fat cottage
		  cheese
		1 (4-oz) apple
			Fast-food meal:
			1 garden salad with
			1 Tbsp regular salad
			  dressing
			1 single hamburger
			8 dried apricots

Dinner	1/2 cup cauliflower with
	1/4 cup garbanzo beans with
	1/2 cup canned or fresh
	  tomatoes sauteed with
	2 tsp olive oil
	Served over
	1/2 cup Curry Couscous
	  (p. 32)
	2 small broiled chicken legs
	1 cup fat-free milk
	1/2 small mango, sliced
		1 cup napa cabbage,
		  stir-fried with
		1/2 cup bean sprouts and
		1 tsp sesame oil and soy
		  sauce
		1 cup Asian Scallop
		  Fettucine (1 cup pasta,
		  3 oz scallops) (p. 49)
		1 cup fat-free milk
		1/2 cup canned or fresh
		  pineapple
			1 cup green salad with
			2 Tbsp reduced-fat salad
			  dressing
			1/2 serving Chicken
			  with Tricolor Peppers
			  (p. 218) over
			2/3 cup brown rice
			1/2 cup fat-free milk
			1 serving Pears Baked
			  with White Wine
			  (p. 149)

	Day 4	Day 5	Day 6
Breakfast	1/2 cup oatmeal with 2 Tbsp raisins 1 cup fat-free milk 1/2 whole-wheat English muffin 1 tsp margarine	1 poached egg on 1 slice raisin bread with 1 tsp margarine 1 cup cream of wheat with 1 tsp margarine 1 1/4 cup whole strawberries (Egg and 1 starch substitutes for 1 milk.)	1/2 cup All Bran with extra fiber 1/2 cup bran flakes 1 small banana 1 cup fat-free milk
Lunch	2 slices whole-wheat bread toasted with 1 oz part-skim cheese melted on each slice of bread topped with Slices of tomato 2 small plums	1 1/4 cups Chicken, Spinach, and Shell Soup (p. 51) (leftovers from last night) 3/4 oz whole-wheat crackers 1 (4-oz) apple	Fast-food meal: 2 slices of thin-crust pizza with red peppers, mushrooms, and onions 1 cup green salad with 1 Tbsp reduced-fat dressing 3 dates (from home)
Dinner	1 cup green salad with 1 Tbsp regular salad dressing 1 1/4 cups Chicken, Spinach, and Shell Soup (p. 51) 1 whole-wheat dinner roll topped with Caramelized Onions (p. 104) 1 cup fat-free milk 1 orange, quartered	1 cup steamed broccoli with 1 tsp margarine 1 serving Teriyaki Tofu Kabobs (p. 196) on 1/2 cup brown rice 1 cup fat-free milk 1/2 pear (4 oz)	3/4 cup Green Beans with Tomatoes and Herbs (p. 105) 6-oz baked potato with 2 Tbsp low-fat cottage cheese 2 oz Teriyaki Glazed Tuna (p. 202) 2 small vanilla sandwich cookies 1/2 cup unsweetened applesauce

	Day 7	Day 8	Day 9
Breakfast	1/2 cup farina with 2 Tbsp raisins 1 cup fat-free milk 1 slice rye toast 1 tsp margarine	2 slices of whole bagel cut in thirds with 1 Tbsp reduced-fat cream cheese 3/4 cup nonfat yogurt with 1/2 cup canned peaches	1 Blueberry Lemon Muffin (p. 132) 3/4 cup nonfat yogurt over 1 cup cubed papaya
Lunch	1 cup sliced cucumbers with 1 tsp olive oil 1 serving Spanish Black Bean Soup (p. 63) 1 oz part-skim cheese on 1/3 oz whole-wheat crackers 1/2 cup canned fruit cocktail	1 cup Arugula and Watercress Salad (p. 116) 2 slices whole-wheat bread with 2 oz smoked turkey and mustard 2 fresh apricots	1 (6–7") whole-wheat pita pocket stuffed with 1/2 cup canned salmon mixed with 1 Tbsp reduced-fat mayonnaise and 1 tsp relish and 1 tsp red onion Tomato slices and alfalfa sprouts 1 (4-oz) apple
Dinner	1/2 cup steamed green beans 1 serving Stir-fry Fish (p. 209) 1 cup fat-free milk 3/4 cup blueberries	1 serving Colorful Lentil Salad (p. 58) served on 1 cup green salad 2 1/2 oz barbecued chicken legs 3 gingersnaps 2 small tangerines	1 cup Soy Kale (p. 115) 1 serving Glazed Parsnips (p. 81) 1 medium ear of corn-on-the-cob with 1 tsp margarine 2 oz roast pork tenderloin 1 cup fat-free milk 1/2 grapefruit

	Day 10	Day 11	Day 12
Breakfast	1/2 cup cooked oat bran with 2 Tbsp dried cranberries 1 slice whole-wheat toast with 1 tsp margarine 1 cup fat-free milk	1 frozen waffle with 2 Tbsp light table syrup (replaces fruit) 1 cup fat-free milk	2 slices whole-wheat bread 1 scrambled egg 1/2 cup grits 1 tsp margarine 1 orange, quartered (Egg and 1 starch substitutes for 1 milk.)
Lunch	3/4 cup Mexican Bean Salad (p. 61) topped with 2 oz tuna fish 1/3 oz whole-wheat crackers 1/2 pear (4 oz)	1 cup green salad with 2 Tbsp reduced-fat salad dressing 1 Chicken Fettucine frozen entree 4 dried apple rings	2 oz Oriental Turkey Salad (p. 222) on 2 slices of whole-wheat bread and Lettuce and tomato slices 1 1/4 cups watermelon cubes
Dinner	1/2 cup steamed green beans 1/2 cup cooked couscous 2 oz lamb from Spiced Lamb Stew (p. 227) 1 cup fat-free milk 1/2 cup fruit cocktail	1 cup steamed asparagus 1 cup linguini topped with 2 Tbsp Pesto (p. 52) and 2 1/2 oz grilled scallops 1/2 cup sugar-free pudding over 1 cup raspberries	1/2 cup Broccoli with Sesame Seeds and Scallions (p. 108) 1 cup butternut squash with 1 tsp margarine 2 oz Chinese Ginger Salmon (p. 199) 1 cup fat-free milk 1 frozen fruit juice bar

	Day 13	Day 14
Breakfast	1 fat-free granola bar 1 cup fat-free milk 1 medium peach	1 bran muffin with 2 Tbsp reduced-fat 　cream cheese 1 cup cubed honeydew 　melon 3/4 cup nonfat yogurt
Lunch	1 cup split pea soup 　(canned) 3/4 oz whole-wheat 　crackers with 2 oz part-skim cheese 1 kiwi	1 1/3 cups Black Bean 　Jicama Salad (p. 62) topped with 2 oz cubed ham 2 small tangerines
Dinner	2 cups green salad with 2 Tbsp regular salad 　dressing 1 serving Seafood Kabobs 　(p. 208) over 1 cup couscous with 1 tsp margarine 1/3 cup nonfat yogurt	1 cup steamed 　cauliflower 1 serving Foil Roasted 　Herb Potatoes (p. 74) 1 serving Grilled 　Chicken Breast with 　Fruit Salsa (p. 219) 1 cup fat-free milk

Two Weeks of Menus for 1,600–1,800 Calorie Range

Breakfast: 57 g carbohydrate/4 Carbohydrate Choices/2 Starch, 1 Fruit, 1 Milk

Lunch: 70 g carbohydrate/4 Carbohydrate Choices/2 Starch, 2 Vegetable, 2 Fruit, 2 Meat

Dinner: 82 g carbohydrate/5 Carbohydrate Choices/3 Starch, 2 Vegetable, 1 Fruit, 1 Milk, 3 Meat

	Day 1	Day 2	Day 3
Breakfast	1 cup oatmeal with 2 Tbsp raisins 1 cup fat-free milk	2/3 cup Spoon Size Shredded Wheat 1/2 cup fat-free milk 1/3 cup nonfat yogurt with 3/4 cup whole strawberries	1 Blueberry Lemon Muffin (p. 132) with 2 tsp margarine 1/2 large grapefruit 1 cup fat-free milk
Lunch	1 cup pre-cut carrots dipped in 2 Tbsp reduced-fat salad dressing 1 6–7″ whole-wheat pita pocket stuffed with 1/2 cup tuna fish made with 2 Tbsp reduced-fat mayonnaise and lettuce and tomato 1 cup cubed honeydew melon with 1 cup cubed cantaloupe	2 cups green salad with 2 Tbsp reduced-fat salad dressing 1 cup Butternut Squash and Pear Soup (p. 82) 2 oz Cheddar cheese 1/3 oz whole-wheat crackers 1 large 8 oz apple	2 servings Orange and Kiwi Salad (p. 142) 2 slices whole-wheat bread 1 oz Swiss cheese 1 oz turkey with 1 Tbsp reduced-fat mayonnaise and lettuce and tomato
Dinner	1 cup green salad with 1/4 cup cold green peas with 2 Tbsp reduced-fat salad dressing 1/2 cup steamed asparagus with 1 tsp margarine 1/2 cup Lemon Raisin Barley and Brown Rice (p. 30) 3 oz broiled lamb chops 1 cup fat-free milk 1 1/4 cups whole strawberries over 1/2 cup strawberry ice cream (regular)	1 cup green salad with 1/2 cup croutons 2 Tbsp regular salad dressing 1 cup Pasta Primavera (p. 45) with 2 oz grilled chicken breast sliced on top of pasta 3/4 cup nonfat yogurt with 1/2 cubed mango	1 Quinoa Stuffed Pepper (p. 34) 1 whole-wheat dinner roll with 1 tsp margarine 3 1/2 oz grilled flank steak 1/2 cup canned plums 3 gingersnaps

	Day 4	Day 5	Day 6

Breakfast	1 cup Wheatena with
	1/2 cup fat-free milk
	1/3 cup nonfat yogurt with
	1 cup raspberries
		1 fried egg with
		1 oz of part-skim Swiss
		  cheese melted
		2 slices whole-wheat bread
		1/2 cup grits with
		1 tsp margarine
		1/2 grapefruit
		(Egg and 1 starch
		  substitutes for 1 milk.)
			1 cup bran flakes
			2 Tbsp dried cranberries
			1 cup fat-free milk

Lunch	1 1/2 cups minestrone
	  soup (canned)
	2 cups green salad with
	1 oz cubed smoked turkey
	  with
	2 Tbsp regular salad
	  dressing
	1 1/2 cups fresh pineapple
		1/2 cup tomato juice
		3/4 cup Almond Pesto
		  White Bean with
		  Vegetable (p. 56)
		  topped with
		2 oz/1/2 cup canned
		  salmon
		3 large dried figs
			2 cups green salad with
			2 Tbsp regular salad
			  dressing
			1 1/4 cups Curried Cauli-
			  flower Soup (p. 112)
			1/3 oz whole-wheat
			  crackers
			1/2 cup low-fat cottage
			  cheese
			8 oz apple cider or juice

Dinner	1 cup Cheese Polenta (p. 40)
	1 cup steamed summer
	  squash and diced onions
	  with
	1 tsp margarine
	3 1/2 oz barbecue chicken
	  breast
	1 slice (1/12th) angel food
	  cake with
	1 1/4 cups whole
	  strawberries, sliced and
	4 Tbsp whipped cream
		1 cup steamed pea pods
		  with
		1 tsp margarine
		1 cup Wild Rice Salad
		  (p. 37)
		3 oz Seared Sesame
		  Tuna with Orange
		  Glaze (p. 201)
		3/4 cup nonfat yogurt
		  with
		1/2 small banana
			1 cup steamed cabbage
			  with
			1 tsp margarine
			2/3 cup baked beans
			3 oz crab meat or
			  steamed crab with
			  cocktail sauce
			1 whole-wheat dinner
			  roll with
			1 tsp margarine
			1 cup fat-free milk
			1/2 cup Blueberries with
			  Almond Cream (p. 131)

	Day 7	Day 8	Day 9
Breakfast	1 cup cream of wheat with 1/2 cup fat-free milk 1 tsp margarine 1/3 cup nonfat yogurt with 1/2 cup canned peaches	1 Blueberry Lemon Muffin (p. 132) with 1 tsp margarine 1 cup fat-free milk 1/2 grapefruit	2 slices of whole bagel cut in thirds 1 tsp margarine 2 tsp no sugar jelly or jam 3/4 cup nonfat yogurt 1/2 cup canned mandarin oranges
Lunch	Chef salad: 2 cups green salad 1 oz cubed chicken or turkey 1 diced hard-boiled egg 2 Tbsp raisins 3 Tbsp regular salad dressing 1 cup reduced-calorie cranberry juice	1 serving Healthy Coleslaw (p. 113) 2 slices whole-wheat bread 1 oz ham 1 oz cheese 1 Tbsp reduced-fat mayonnaise 2 Clementines	2 slices thin-crust pizza topped with sliced tomato, green pepper, and pineapple 2 cups green salad with 2 Tbsp regular salad dressing 2 oranges
Dinner	1/2 cup steamed broccoli with lemon 1 tsp margarine 1 serving Confetti Rice and Beans (p. 39) 1 2″ cube corn bread 3-oz pork chop 3/4 cup nonfat yogurt with 1 cup raspberries	1 serving Penne Pasta with Balsamic Vinaigrette (p. 46) 3 1/2 oz grilled trout cooked with lemon and olive oil 1 granola bar crushed over 1 small sliced banana	1 cup steamed cabbage with 1 tsp margarine 1 serving Sweet Potato Fries (p. 71) 3/4 cup green peas with 1 tsp margarine 3 oz baked ham 1 cup fat-free milk 1/2 cup canned pineapple

	Day 10	Day 11	Day 12
Breakfast	1 English muffin 1 egg scrambled 1/2 cup oatmeal 2 tsp margarine 1/2 cup calcium-fortified orange juice	1 bran muffin with 2 Tbsp reduced-fat cream cheese 1 cup nonfat yogurt with 1 1/4 cups whole strawberries, sliced	3/4 cup/1 serving Strawberry Almond Shake (p. 134) 1/2 cup fat-free milk 1/2 cup fat-free granola cereal
Lunch	2 cups green salad with 2 Tbsp regular salad dressing 1 serving White Bean Chili (p. 64) with 1 oz shredded part-skim cheddar cheese 2 small nectarines	Fast-food meal: 1 regular hamburger 1 large salad with 3 Tbsp salad dressing 6 prunes (from home)	1 cup green salad with 1/2 cup cold steamed beets (leftovers) with 2 Tbsp regular salad dressing 1 1/4 cups Shrimp and Corn Bisque (p. 171) 1 whole-wheat dinner roll with 1 oz part-skim cheese 1 apple (4 oz)
Dinner	1/2 cup marinated artichoke hearts 1 serving Crunchy Shrimp and Broccoli Stir-fry (p. 206) 3/4 cup pasta 1 serving Just Peachy Crisp (p. 270)	1 cup steamed beets with 1 tsp margarine 1 serving Shrimp and Bean Skillet (p. 67) 3/4 cup brown rice with 1 tsp margarine 1 cup fat-free milk 1/2 cup fresh or canned fruit cup	1 cup green salad with 1/4 cup chickpeas with 2 Tbsp regular salad dressing 1 serving Oven-dried Tomatoes, Garlic, and Pasta (p. 48) topped with 3 oz turkey sausage 3/4 cup nonfat yogurt 3/4 cup blueberries

	Day 13	Day 14

Breakfast	1/2 cup Cheerios
	1/2 cup All Bran with
	   Fiber
	1 cup fat-free milk
	1 small banana
		2 (4″) pancakes with
		1 tsp margarine and
		2 Tbsp light syrup
		3/4 cup nonfat yogurt
		   with
		1/2 cup cubed mango

Lunch	2 slices whole-wheat
	   bread
	1/2 cup (2 oz) tuna with
	1 Tbsp regular
	   mayonnaise topped with
	lettuce and tomato
	1 cup pre-cut carrots
	1 large apple (8 oz)
		2 cups green salad with
		2 Tbsp regular salad
		   dressing
		1 cup angel hair pasta with
		2 Tbsp Pesto (p. 52)
		   topped with
		2 oz Parmesan cheese
		6 dates

Dinner	1/2 cup Zucchini Marinara
	   (p. 106)
	1 cup mashed potatoes
	   with
	2 tsp margarine
	3 oz Crispy Fish Fillets
	   (p. 212)
	1 cup fat-free milk
	2 Clementines
		3 oz chicken and 1/2 cup
		   of stuffing from Wild
		   Rice Sun-dried Cherry
		   Stuffed Chicken
		   (p. 216)
		1 cup winter squash with
		1 tsp margarine
		1 whole-wheat dinner
		   roll with
		1 tsp margarine
		3/4 cup nonfat yogurt
		1 sliced peach

Two Weeks of Menus for 2,000–2,200 Calorie Range

Breakfast: 72 g carbohydrate/5 Carbohydrate Choices/3 Starch, 1 Fruit, 1 Milk

Lunch: 85 g carbohydrate/5 Carbohydrate Choices/3 Starch, 2 Vegetable, 2 Fruit, 3 Meat

Dinner: 86 g carbohydrate/6 Carbohydrate Choices/4 Starch, 2 Vegetable, 1 Fruit, 1 Milk, 3 Meat

	Day 1	Day 2	Day 3
Breakfast	4 Nutty Blueberry Pancakes (p. 31) with 2 Tbsp sugar-free table syrup 3/4 cup nonfat yogurt with 1 medium peach, sliced	1 cup raisin bran flakes 1 cup fat-free milk 1/2 cup calcium-fortified orange juice 1 slice whole-wheat toast with 1 tsp margarine	1 cup cooked oat bran cereal with 1/2 cup fat-free milk 1 slice whole-wheat toast with 1 tsp margarine 3/4 cup blueberries 1/3 cup nonfat yogurt
Lunch	3/4 cup Mango Chicken Salad (p. 140) on 2 cups of salad greens with 2 Tbsp regular salad dressing 8 slices melba toast 1 kiwi	2 cups green salad with 2 Tbsp regular salad dressing 1 Apple Sandwich (p. 146) with 2 oz ham made on 2 slices of regular whole-wheat bread 2 oz potato chips 1/2 cup unsweetened applesauce	3/4 cup Fall Spinach Salad (p. 114) topped with 3 oz tuna fish or cubed chicken 1 6–7″ whole-wheat pita pocket with 2 tsp margarine 1 (8-oz) pear
Dinner	1 cup green salad with 1 Tbsp regular salad dressing 3/4 cup Wild Rice Pilaf (p. 38) 1 cup corn with 1 tsp margarine 3 oz grilled bluefish with 1 tsp olive oil and lemon 3/4 cup nonfat yogurt 1/2 cup orange and grapefruit sections	2 cups green salad topped with 1/2 cup croutons 1 Festive Sweet Potato (p. 72) 3/4 cup green peas with 1 tsp margarine 3 oz grilled chicken 1 cup fat-free milk	1 cup green salad topped with 3/4 cup mandarin oranges and 2 Tbsp regular salad dressing 1 cup Fusilli with Sage and Peppers (p. 44) topped with 2 oz turkey sausage and 1 oz grated Parmesan cheese 1 slice whole-wheat bread with 1 tsp margarine 1 cup fat-free milk

	Day 4	Day 5	Day 6

Breakfast	1/2 cup oatmeal with
	1 tsp margarine
	2 Tbsp raisins
	1 cup fat-free milk
	1 whole-wheat English
	   muffin
	2 tsp margarine
		1 fried egg
		1 oz Canadian bacon
		2 slices whole-wheat
		   bread with
		1 tsp margarine
		1/2 cup grits with
		1 tsp margarine
		1/2 grapefruit
			2 frozen waffles with
			1 tsp margarine
			2 Tbsp light table syrup
			3/4 cup nonfat yogurt
			1 1/4 cup whole
			   strawberries

Lunch	1 cup pre-cut carrots
	   dipped in
	2 Tbsp regular salad
	   dressing
	4 oz Red Grape and
	   Turkey Salad (p. 148) in
	1 6–7″ whole-wheat pita
	   pocket stuffed with
	1 cup lettuce
	1 medium banana
		2 cups cut up raw
		   vegetables (red
		   peppers, broccoli,
		   mushrooms) dipped in
		2 Tbsp salad dressing
		1 serving French Bread
		   Pizza frozen entree
		1 (8-oz) apple
			1 cup celery sticks with
			2 Tbsp regular salad
			   dressing
			1 Vegetable Burrito (p. 80)
			3 oz grated Monterey
			   Jack cheese in or on
			   burrito
			4 Tbsp raisins

Dinner	1 cup Orange and Fennel
	   Salad (p. 135)
	1 cup Polenta (p. 40) with
	1 tsp margarine
	1 cup acorn squash with
	1 tsp margarine
	3 oz Seared Salmon with
	   Asparagus and Green
	   Onion (p. 200)
	1 cup fat-free milk
		2 cup green salad with
		2 Tbsp regular salad
		   dressing
		2 servings Cranberry
		   Rice (p. 42)
		3 1/2 oz baked ham
		1 cup fat-free milk
		4″ brownie (not frosted)
			1/2 cup pea pods stir-
			   fried in
			1 tsp olive oil and soy
			   sauce
			1 serving Asian Noodle
			   Salad (p. 47) with
			3 oz grilled chicken
			   breast sliced on top
			3/4 cup nonfat yogurt
			1 medium peach, sliced

	Day 7	Day 8	Day 9
Breakfast	1 whole bagel with 2 Tbsp reduced-fat cream cheese 3/4 cup nonfat yogurt 1 cup papaya cubes	3/4 cup multi bran Chex 1/2 cup wheat bran flakes 1 cup fat-free milk 1 small banana	1 Dunkin Donut Oat Bran muffin 1/2 cup orange juice 1 cup fat-free milk
Lunch	2 cups green salad with 1/2 cup kidney beans with 2 Tbsp regular salad dressing 1 serving Strawberry Peach Soup 1 whole-wheat dinner roll with 1 tsp margarine 2 Fig Newtons 1 small plum	1/2 cup cold beets Lettuce and tomato slices 2 slices whole-wheat bread 3 oz canned salmon mixed with 1 Tbsp regular mayonnaise 2 tangerines	1 cup carrots pre-cut dipped in 2 Tbsp regular salad dressing 1 serving Bow Tie Pasta with Sun-dried Tomato Pesto and White Beans (p. 57) (leftover from last night) topped with 3 oz crumbled feta cheese 1 (8-oz) pear
Dinner	1 cup spinach with 1 tsp margarine 1/4 recipe Chive Corn Pudding (p. 79) 1 2 1/2″ biscuit 1 2-oz broiled pork chop 1/3 cup nonfat yogurt with 3/4 cup blueberries	1/2 cup steamed zucchini with 1 tsp margarine 1 serving Bow Tie Pasta with Sun Dried Tomato Pesto and White Beans (p. 57) 2″ cube corn bread 3 oz sautéed flounder with 1 tsp olive oil and lemon 1 cup fat-free buttermilk 1 1/4 cups watermelon cubes	1 cup green salad with 1 Tbsp regular salad dressing 1/2 Spinach Sauté with Mushrooms (p. 117) 1 1/2 cups spaghetti topped with 1 serving Shrimp Scampi (p. 211) 1 whole-wheat dinner roll 1 cup fat-free milk 1/2 cup canned peaches

	Day 10	Day 11	Day 12
Breakfast	1 cup cream of wheat 1/2 whole-wheat English muffin with 1 tsp margarine 1 cup fat-free milk 1/2 grapefruit	1 poached egg on 1 slice raisin bread with 1 tsp margarine 1 cup oatmeal 3/4 cup nonfat yogurt 3/4 cup blueberries	3/4 cup bran flakes 1 cup corn flakes 1 cup fat-free milk 2 Tbsp dried cranberries
Lunch	1 6″ roast beef and provolone cheese sub sandwich (from sub shop) with lettuce, tomato, onion, and hot peppers with mustard and 1 Tbsp regular mayonnaise 1 (8-oz) apple	1 1/2 cups Indian Bean Salad (p. 61) topped with 3 oz grilled chicken 34 small grapes	3 oz Chicken Salad 64 Ways (p. 220) served on 1 cup greens, sliced cucumbers, and tomatoes 1 1/2 oz whole-wheat crackers 2 tangerines
Dinner	2 cups green salad with 2 Tbsp regular salad dressing 1 serving Angel Hair with Feta and Capers (p. 50) 1 whole-wheat dinner roll with Roasted Garlic (p. 103) 3 oz grilled shrimp 1 cup fat-free milk 1/2 cup canned apricots	1 serving Cioppino (p. 207) 2 slices Italian bread with 2 tsp olive oil 1 cup fat-free milk 1 slice Old-Fashioned Spiced Banana Bread (p. 269) 1 1/4 cups whole strawberries	1 serving Pasta Fagioli (p. 59) 1 slice whole-wheat bread with 1 tsp margarine 3 oz grilled flank steak 1 cup fat-free milk 1 cup cantaloupe cubes

	Day 13	Day 14
Breakfast	1 3/4 cups Strawberry Almond Shake (p. 134) 1 fat-free granola bar	1 whole bagel with 2 tsp margarine and 2 tsp low-sugar jelly or jam 1 cup fat-free milk 1/2 cup fruit cocktail (fresh or canned)
Lunch	1 serving Middle Eastern Tuna Salad (p. 203) in 1 1/2 (6–7″) whole-wheat pita pocket with 1 Tbsp regular mayonnaise 1 kiwi sliced with 1 orange sliced	Fast-food meal: 1 grilled chicken sandwich with lettuce and tomato 1 small order French fries (split) 1 garden salad with 1 Tbsp regular salad dressing 1/2 cup applesauce with 2 Tbsp raisins
Dinner	1 cup reduced-calorie cranberry juice 2 cups green salad with 1/2 cup croutons with 2 Tbsp regular salad dressing 1 serving Red Bean Creole (p. 65) topped with 3 oz turkey sausage 1 cup fat-free milk	2 cups green salad with 2 Tbsp regular salad dressing 1 1/2 cups fettucine noodles with 1/2 cup Marinara Sauce (p. 52) with 3 1/2 oz ground hamburger mixed into sauce 5 vanilla wafers 8 dried apricots

	Desire weight loss*	Many older women	Women, older adults	Larger women, older men	Children, teen girls, active women, most men	Teen boys, active men
Calorie level	About 1200	About 1400	About 1600	About 1800	About 2200	About 2800
Calorie range	1200–1500	1300–1600	1400–1700	1600–1900	1800–2300	2200–2800
Carbohydrate (g)	180	180	195	210	240	300
Carbohydrate Choices	12	12	13	14	16	20
Grains, beans, and starchy vegetables	6	6	6	7	9	11
Vegetables	3	3	3	4	4	5
Fruits	3	3	3	3	3	4
Milk†	2	2	2-3	2-3	2-3	2-3
Meats	2 (4 oz)	2 (4 oz)	2 (5 oz)	2 (5 oz)	2 (6 oz)	3 (7 oz)
Fats g/servings (based on 30% of calories as fat)	40/4	47/5	54/6	60/7	74/9	93/12

* Some older women and men who are small in stature and sedentary may need to eat no more than 1200 calories to lose weight. At 1200 calories, you may need a vitamin and mineral supplement that provides 100% of the Daily Value to meet your nutrition needs.

†Teenagers, young adults to age 24, and women who are pregnant or breastfeeding and adults older than 50 need 1200 mg of calcium each day. Adults younger than 50 need 1000 mg of calcium per day. Each cup of milk or yogurt contains about 300 mg of calcium. Other sources of calcium are calcium-fortified orange juice, other dairy products, and dark-green, leafy vegetables. If you do not get sufficient calcium from the foods you eat, talk to your health care provider about taking a calcium supplement to meet your requirements for calcium. Each serving of milk is equivalent to about 12 grams of carbohydrate or roughly 1 carbohydrate choice.

To develop more specific and individualized recommendations about the amount of carbohydrate you should eat at meals and snacks, work with a dietitian or diabetes educator with expertise in diabetes.

How to Find a Dietitian

Many people find that balancing food with medication and activity is the most challenging part of diabetes management. You don't have to face this challenge alone!

A dietitian with expertise in diabetes can be an invaluable partner. Here are three ways to find a dietitian:

- American Diabetes Association's Recognized Diabetes Education Programs.

  All these programs have at least one dietitian. Find programs in your area by calling 800-DIABETES (800-342-2383). Via the Internet go to **www.diabetes.org/education/eduprogram.asp.**

- Find a diabetes educator who is a dietitian by calling the American Association of Diabetes Educators at 800-TEAMUP4 (832-6874). Via the internet, go to **www.diabeteseducator.org** and go to Find a Diabetes Educator.

- Ask your doctor for a referral.

Who Pays?

Traditionally, nutrition counseling has not been covered by health plans. That's changing. To date, 42 states have passed legislation mandating that private insurance policies and managed care plans, which must follow that state's laws, cover nutrition counseling for residents with diabetes. Contact your American Diabetes Association by phone (1-800-DIABETES) or the Internet (**www.diabetes.org**) to see if your state has a law.

While the content of these laws varies widely, most laws cover people with type 1, type 2, or gestational diabetes. Most of the laws specifically mention "medical nutrition therapy" as a covered service. However, these laws cover only about 30% of people. The other 70% of the population are covered by Medicare, employer health plans, or they are without health care coverage.

If you have Medicare part B (services outside of the hospital), you should be able to get your nutrition counseling covered within an ADA Recognized Diabetes Education Program or as of January 2002 by a registered dietitian. However, criteria for this counseling do exist. Call your local Medicare office listed in the Government pages of your phone book or go to Medicare's Internet site, **www.medicare.gov**.

If you have health coverage through a large employer, you may or may not be able to get nutrition counseling covered. Large employer group health plans are generally not covered by the state laws mentioned above. Call your health plan and ask if they cover this benefit. Ask if you need a referral from your doctor. Health plans often require a written referral to document "medical necessity." Also ask if there are certain dietitians you must go to in order to have your insurer cover the sessions and how many sessions they cover.

You may well have to be your own advocate to get nutrition counseling covered by your health plan. A letter from your doctor and dietitian may help, along with a letter written by you stating how your diabetes control has improved with nutrition counseling. If you can show them you are saving them money, they like that. For example, maybe you now take less medication or you have not been to the emergency room in the past six months.

If you don't have a health plan that covers nutrition counseling, or you have no health plan at all, then the choice is yours whether to reach into your pocket and pay for nutrition counseling. It will be money well spent and not that expensive relative to medications, hospitalizations, or even a restaurant meal. A nutrition counseling session varies widely from about $50 to $150. Some dietitians offer a package that includes a number of sessions.

The Food Label

Helps You Make Healthy Choices

Today the supermarket is a virtual warehouse of nutrition information. The current Nutrition Facts panel that is on nearly every packaged food is one of the best sources—and it's free. No charge for reading the large or fine print, or for comparing the numbers on several different labels. It's the Government's way of helping you play Sherlock Holmes as you strive to eat the healthiest way you can.

THE OLD AND THE NEW

Before 1994 the nutrition labeling of foods was sparse and to a large extent provided voluntarily by manufacturers.

In 1994 the so-called "new food label" premiered. It reflected the new food labeling law enforced by the Food and Drug Administration (FDA) and U.S. Department of Agriculture (USDA). The huge change was intended to clear up confusion fostered by the old label, to help people choose healthy foods, and to offer an incentive to food companies to improve the nutritional qualities of the foods they produce. Now the food label is the most popular read in the supermarket—well, maybe after the National Enquirer.

Key features of the current food label:

- Now almost all foods give you Nutrition Facts.

- The same easy-to-read format must be used on most products, unless the label is too small.

- Serving sizes used by manufacturers must be the same within product categories to allow you to do a fair comparison. Servings are also closer to what is reasonable and usual. In the old days, manufacturers could set their own serving size, so if a manufacturer wanted its product to look as if it had fewer calories or less fat, it could make the serving size very small. Not anymore! All the cracker manufacturers, for example, have to use the same serving size, and you can easily compare the fat content of different crackers.

- Nutrition claims that brag about a food's nutrient content—such as "light," "low-fat," and "high-fiber"—are defined by the governing authorities, not the food manufacturers.

- Health claims that boast about the food's health benefits are defined by the governing authorities.

- Manufacturers of fruit drinks must state on the label the percentage of fruit juice in the drink.

297

WHAT HAS A LABEL

Almost all packaged and processed foods have food labels. A few exceptions are very small packages on which the information doesn't fit; bulk foods such as cereals or nuts sold from barrels; foods with next to no nutrients, such as coffee, tea, spices, and herbs.

A voluntary program was set up to have supermarkets provide nutrition information for many raw foods. Therefore in many grocery stores, you can get nutrition information on:

• 20 most frequently eaten raw fruits, vegetables, and fish (under FDA's voluntary point-of-purchase nutrition information program)

• 45 best-selling cuts of meat (under USDA's program).

WHAT'S ON THE LABEL

Instant Oatmeal

① **Nutrition Facts**
② Serving Size: 1 Packet (35g) [Note: This is 2 starch exchanges]
Servings per Container: 10

	AMOUNT PER SERVING
Calories 130	
③ Calories from Fat 15	

	% DAILY VALUE
④ **Total Fat** 1.5g	2%
Saturated Fat 0.5g	2%
Polyunsaturated Fat 0.5g	
Monounsaturated Fat 0.5g	
Cholesterol 0mg	0%
⑤ **Sodium** 170mg	7%
⑥ **Total Carbohydrate** 27g	9%
Dietary Fiber 3g	11%
Soluble Fiber 1g	
⑦ Sugars 12g	
Protein 3g	0%

	% DAILY VALUE
⑧ Vitamin A	20%
Vitamin C	0%
Calcium	10%
Iron	20%
⑨ Thiamin	20%
Riboflavin	20%
Niacin	20%
Vitamin B6	20%
Folic Acid	20%
Phosphorus	8%

*Percent Daily Values are based on a 2,000 calorie diet. Your daily values may be higher or lower depending on your calorie needs.

⑩	Calories	2,000	2,500
Total Fat	Less than	65 g	80 g
Sat Fat	Less than	20 g	25 g
Cholesterol	Less than	300 mg	300 mg
Sodium	Less than	2,400 mg	2,400 mg
Total Carbohydrate		300 g	375 g
Dietary Fiber	25	g 30	g
Calorie per gram:			
Fat 9	Carbohydrate 4		Protein 4

① Nutrition Facts

Manufacturers are required to use this header and the format below it unless their product meets exemptions. The law requires manufacturers to use certain type size, style, spacing, and contrast so the label is easy to read.

② Serving Size

- All the nutrition information in the label is based on the amount of food in one serving.

- The serving size must be expressed in both common household ("1 packet") and metric measures ("35 g").

- Servings for 139 categories of foods were established by the FDA and must be followed by manufacturers. These "reference amounts" are based on the amount of that food that people usually eat.

One Serving Only

Rules for foods packaged as individual servings have changed as well. If the contents of a package are less than 2 times the amount of the reference serving, the item must be called one serving. The nutrition information must be given for the entire package (as 1 serving). For example, the standard serving size for a carbonated beverage is 8 fluid ounces, but the standard can is 12 ounces. Twelve ounces is less than double the standard serving. Therefore, it must be called one serving and the nutrition facts must be given for all 12 ounces.

Not Always a Match

The FDA reference serving size for products may or may not be the same as those in various diabetes meal planning tools. Compare the reference serving on the food label with the serving size in the diabetes meal planning approach you use. For some foods, they are the same. For example, 1/2 cup canned beans is one Diabetes Food Pyramid serving, one Exchange, and one food label serving. But for other foods, the food label serving size is different from the exchange:

Food	Food Label Serving	Diabetes Serving or Exchange
Butter or margarine (regular stick)	1 Tbsp	1 tsp
Fruit juice	8 oz (1 cup)	depends on juice: 1/3 or 1/2 cup
Vegetable juice	8 oz (1 cup)	4 oz (1/2 cup)
Salad dressing (regular)	2 Tbsp	1 Tbsp

If the serving sizes are the same, then it's a snap to interpret the nutrition information. If they're different, you need to do the math. For example, say you choose to use 1 tsp of regular margarine, which is 1 fat exchange. If you want to know the nutrient counts (for example, how many grams of saturated fat you're eating), you need to divide the numbers on the Nutrition Facts by 3, because 1 tablespoon is a "label" serving, and there are 3 teaspoons in 1 tablespoon. If you want to use 1 Tbsp, you need to count it as 3 fat exchanges.

③ Calories from Fat, Total Fat, Saturated Fat, Cholesterol

See Focus on Fats, p. 159.

④ % Daily Values

The percent of each nutrient that is provided in one serving of the product, based on the daily values for 2,000 calories a day. Two thousand calories is used because it's considered an average calorie intake for adults. However, it may be too low or too high for you. Percent daily value is not on food labels using the simplified format because there's not enough space.

⑤ Sodium

The recommendation for most healthy adults and people with mild to moderate hypertension (high blood pressure) is to consume less than 2,400 mg per day of sodium, and that's the figure the % Daily Value uses. It's recommended that people with hypertension and kidney disease consume less than 2,000 mg per day of sodium.

⑥ Total Carbohydrate

It's the carbohydrate in foods that will your raise blood glucose levels the most and the fastest. Thus, you want to learn how to look at a food label and be able to figure out how to count the grams of carbohydrate into your meal plan.

Look at the Total Carbohydrate, which is the amount in one serving of the food. If you are counting grams of carbohydrate in your approach to meal planning, then just determine how many servings of the food you will eat and the number of grams of carbohydrate that will be.

If you're counting carbohydrate choices or exchanges, you need to know that 1 choice or exchange of carbohydrate contains 15 grams of carbohydrate. It's equal to 1 starch, fruit, or milk serving or exchange. Use this table to figure out how to count the number of grams of carbohydrate on a food label into your food plan.

Total Carbohydrate (grams in one serving)	Count as
0–5 grams	Do not count
6–10 grams	1/2 carbohydrate choice or exchange
11–20 grams	1 carbohydrate choice or serving
21–25 grams	1 1/2 carbohydrate choices or servings
26–35 grams	2 carbohydrate choices or servings

7 Sugars

Sugars are listed on the Nutrition Facts panel as a subcategory of Total Carbohydrate. Most people zero in on that sugars count. Don't! Remember that when it comes to your blood glucose levels, it's the total amount of carbohydrate that matters. Don't pay special attention to the grams of sugars because they have already been counted as part of the grams of Total Carbohydrate.

The sugars can be from two origins:

• Natural sugars, such as milk sugar or fruit sugar

• Added sugars, such as corn syrup, high-fructose corn syrup, and honey

You can't look at the grams of sugars and know whether the sugars are from natural or added sources. You can get a sense of the sources of sugars by reading the ingredients.

No-Added-Sugar Applesauce

Nutrition Facts
Serving Size: 1/2 cup

	AMOUNT PER SERVING
Calories	50

Total Carbohydrate 15g
   Sugars 11g

Ingredients: Apples, water. (That's all.)

Sweetened Applesauce

Nutrition Facts
Serving Size: 1/2 cup

	AMOUNT PER SERVING
Calories	90

Total Carbohydrate 23g
   Sugars 18g

Ingredients: Apples, corn syrup, high fructose corn syrup, sugar

8 Vitamins and Minerals

The label must list the percent of the Reference Daily Intake (RDI) for vitamin A, vitamin C, calcium, and iron provided in a serving of the food.

If you want to know how much of a vitamin or mineral a food contains as a number rather than percent, make a list from the table below and keep it with you. Look at a label and calculate the amount you will get per serving of the product.

For example, if you look at the label of fat-free milk, you see that a serving has 30% calcium. The RDI for calcium is 1000 milligrams, so you know that the milk has about 300 milligrams per 8 ounces. If you're over age 51, your recommended intake is 1,200 mg, so a serving (1 cup) of fat-free milk gives you 25% of your recommended intake.

Reference Daily Intakes/ Daily Values used by FDA	
Vitamin A	5,000 IU
Vitamin C	60 mg
Iron	18 mg
Calcium	1,000 mg
Vitamin D	400 IU
Vitamin E	30 IU

9 Other Vitamins and Minerals

If a nutrition claim is made about other vitamins or minerals, the percent of RDI provided in the food must be on the label. For example, for the claim "One serving provides the day's need for B vitamins," the label must include nutrition information for all the B vitamins. A manufacturer is allowed to voluntarily list the nutrition content for more vitamins and minerals.

10 Daily Values

List of the daily values for selected nutrients for 2,000 and 2,500 calories per day. These two calorie levels are used because an "average" woman needs around 2,000 calories per day and an "average" man needs 2,500. This is mandatory, unless the label is too small.

You may want to carry your own personalized list of daily values (for example, how many grams of fat you want to consume in a day). Put these numbers on a small piece of paper, and keep them in your wallet. Refer to your daily values when you want to see how particular foods will or will not fit into your meal plan.

When judging the percent of daily value, think how you will use the food. Is it a snack? If it gives you 20% of the amount of fat you should have in a day, 20% is high. However, if you're going to use the food as a main course, 20% is a reasonable amount.

Other required items on package:

- Name of food
- Manufacturer's name and address
- Net weight of contents in package
- Ingredient list: Lists the ingredients in the food in descending order of quantity by weight.

Label Formats: Different From the Rest

The nutrition labeling regulations allow several different label formats.

- When the food contains insignificant amounts of seven or more of the mandatory nutrients and total calories, the product can have a different format. Insignificant is defined as zero or less than 1 gram.

Five "core nutrients" must be listed: total calories, total fat, total carbohydrate, protein, and sodium. They must be listed even if they are present in insignificant amounts. Other nutrients, along with calories from fat, must be shown if they are present in more than insignificant amounts. Some manufacturers will put a note on the label showing what nutrients are not there in a significant quantity, but this is not required.

- When package has less than 12 square inches of available labeling space (about the size of a package of chewing gum), it doesn't have to carry nutrition information unless a nutrient content or health claim is made for the product. However, it must provide an address or telephone number for consumers to obtain the required nutrition information. If manufacturers wish to provide nutrition information on these packages voluntarily, they have two options: 1) present the information in a smaller type size than that required for larger packages, or 2) present the information in a tabular or linear (string) format.

Herb Tea

Nutrition Facts

Serving Size: 1 tea bag (2g)
Servings per Container: 20

	AMOUNT PER SERVING
Calories	0

	% DAILY VALUE
Total Fat 0g	0%
Sodium 0mg	0%
Total Carbohydrate 0g	0%
Sugars 0g	
Protein 0g	0%

- When products have less than 40 square inches of surface area and not enough space for the full vertical format, other formats may be used. Names of dietary components may be abbreviated. All footnotes, except for the statement that % Daily Values are based on 2,000 calories a day, can be omitted. Nutrition information can be placed on other panels readily seen by consumers.

- For products that require preparation before eating, such as macaroni and cheese, or that are usually eaten with one or more additional foods, such as dry cereals with milk, FDA encourages manufacturers to voluntarily provide a second column of nutrition information. The first column, which is mandatory, contains nutrition information for the food as purchased. The second gives information about the food as prepared and eaten.

Raisin and Bran Flakes Cereal

Nutrition Facts
Serving Size: 1 cup or 59g
Servings per Container: About 7

AMOUNT PER SERVING	CEREAL	CEREAL WITH 1/2 CUP VITAMINS A&D FAT-FREE MILK
Calories 190		230
Calories from Fat 15		15
	% DAILY VALUE	
Total Fat 1.5g* 0%		2%
Saturated Fat 0g 0%		0%
Cholesterol 0mg 0%		0%
Sodium 350mg 15%		17%
Total Carbohydrate 45g 15%		17%
Dietary Fiber 8g 32%		32%
Sugars 18g		
Protein 5g 0%		0%
Vitamin A 15%		20%
Vitamin C 0%		2%
Calcium 2%		15%
Iron 25%		25%

* Amount in cereal. One half cup of fat-free milk contributes an additional 40 calories, 65mg sodium, 6g total carbohydrate (6g sugars), and 4g protein.

Nutrition Claims

Food manufacturers may make what is called "a nutrition claim" on a food package. If a nutrition claim is made on the product, the manufacturer must put the statement "see panel for nutrition information" on the front of the package near the nutrition claim. If the claim is about a nutrient that is not required, then that information must be included in the labeling information. For example, if a product states "Provides 1/3 of all vitamins and minerals for which an RDA exists," the data for all those vitamins and minerals must be on the nutrition facts panel. Three categories of nutrient claims exist:

- Absolute claims, such as "low-sodium" or "sugar-free"

- Relative or comparative claims, such as "reduced" or "less"

- Implied claims such as "high in oat bran," which implies it is high in dietary fiber

The following are the currently allowed nutrition claims and their FDA definitions.

Nutrition Claim	Definition
Calorie free	Less than 5 calories per serving
Fat free	Less than 0.5 g per serving
Cholesterol free	Less than 2 mg of cholesterol per serving
Sugar free	Less than 0.5 g sugars per serving
Low fat	Less than 3 g per serving or 3 g per 100 g of main dish
Low saturated fat	1 g or less saturated fat per serving
Low sodium	140 mg or less sodium per serving
Very low sodium	35 mg or less sodium per serving
Reduced calorie	At least 25% fewer calories than regular food
Reduced fat	At least 25% less fat than regular food
Reduced sugars	At least 25% less sugar than regular food
No added sugar, without added sugar, no sugar added	Permitted if no amount of sugars or ingredient that substitutes for sugar is used, contains no fruit juice concentrate or jelly, the label says the food is not low calorie
High fiber	5 g or more per serving
More or added fiber	2.5 g or more per serving than the reference food

Nutrition Claim	Definition
Light or Lite	One-third fewer calories, or half the fat, or half the sodium. If it means light in color or texture, product must state what is light, for example, "light in color," "light brown sugar," or "light and fluffy."
Healthy	Must be low in fat and saturated fat and contain limited amounts of cholesterol and sodium. The sodium levels are 360 mg per serving for individual foods and 480 mg per serving for meal-type products. In addition, if it's a single-item food, it must provide at least 10% of one or more of vitamins A or C, iron, calcium, protein, or fiber. If it's a meal-type product, such as frozen entrees and multi-course frozen dinners, it must provide 10% of two or three of these vitamins or minerals or of protein or fiber, in addition to meeting the other criteria.
Fresh	Can be used only on a food that is raw, has never been frozen or heated, and contains no preservatives
Good source of . . .	Has 10–19% of the Daily Value per serving
Excellent source of . . .	Has 20% of the Daily Value per serving
More	A serving of food, whether altered or not, contains a nutrient that is at least 10% of the Daily Value more than the reference food.
Fortified, added, or enriched	A serving of food that has been altered contains a nutrient that is at least 10% of the Daily Value more than the reference food.
Hi and Lo	These alternative spellings of "high" and "low" and their synonyms are allowed as long as the alternatives are not misleading.
Percent fat-free	Must be a low-fat or a fat-free product. The claim must accurately reflect the amount of fat present in 100 g of the food. Thus, if a food contains 2.5 g fat per 50 g, the claim must be "95% fat-free."
Meals and main dishes	Claims that a meal or main dish is "free" of a nutrient, such as sodium or cholesterol, must meet the same requirements as those for individual foods.

Nutrition Claim	Definition
Lean (Applies to meat, poultry, seafood, and game. Falls within the jurisdiction of the USDA.)	Less than 10 g total fat, less than 4 g saturated fat, and less than 95 mg cholesterol per serving and 100 g
Extra lean	Less than 5 g total fat, less than 2 g saturated fat, and less than 95 mg cholesterol per serving and 100 g

Health Claims

With the new food label came an OK from FDA for manufacturers to make health claims about and on their products. But not just any health claim can be used. To date claims for 12 relationships between a nutrient or a food and the risk of a disease or health condition are allowed. Currently, no health claims are directly related to diabetes.

These claims can be made in several ways:

- through third-party references, such as the National Cancer Institute

- statements

- symbols, such as a heart

- vignettes or descriptions

Whatever way is used, the claim must meet the requirements for authorized health claims. The health claim

- Can't state the degree of risk reduction, such as "Eating this food can reduce your incidence of developing heart disease by X%."

- Can use only the words "may" or "might" in discussing the nutrient or food-disease relationship.

- Must state that other factors play a role in that disease.

- Must be phrased so that consumers can understand the relationship between the nutrient and the disease and the nutrient's importance in relationship to a daily diet.

An example of an appropriate claim is: "While many factors affect heart disease, diets low in saturated fat and cholesterol may reduce the risk of this disease."

Health Claim	Definition
Calcium and osteoporosis	To carry this claim, a food must contain 20% or more of the Daily Value for calcium (200 mg) per serving, have a calcium content that equals or exceeds the food's content of phosphorus, and contain a form of calcium that can be readily absorbed and used by the body. The claim must name the target group most in need of adequate calcium intakes (that is, teens and young adult white and Asian women) and state the need for exercise and a healthy diet. A product that contains 40% or more of the Daily Value for calcium must state on the label that a total dietary intake greater than 200% of the Daily Value for calcium (that is, 2,000 mg or more) has no further known benefit.
Dietary fat and cancer	The food must meet the food label descriptor requirements for "low fat" or, if fish and game meats, for "extra lean."
Saturated fat and cholesterol and coronary heart disease (CHD)	This claim may be used if the food meets the definitions for the descriptors "low saturated fat," "low cholesterol," and "low fat," or, if meat, poultry, seafood, or game, for "extra lean." It may mention the link between reduced risk of CHD and lower saturated fat and cholesterol intakes to lower blood cholesterol levels.
Fiber-containing grain products, fruits, and vegetables and cancer	The food must be or must contain a grain product, fruit, or vegetable and meet the requirements for "low fat," and, without fortification, be a "good source" of dietary fiber. "Good" is 10–19% of the RDI which is 11.5 grams/1,000 calories or 25 grams/2,000 calories.
Fruits, vegetables, and grain products that contain fiber and risk of CHD	To carry this claim, a food must be or must contain fruits, vegetables, and grain products. It also must meet the descriptor requirements for "low saturated fat," "low cholesterol," and "low fat," and contain, without fortification, at least 0.6 g soluble fiber per serving.
Sodium and high blood pressure	The food must meet the requirements for "low-sodium."
Fruits and vegetables and cancer	This claim may be made for fruits and vegetables that meet the requirements for "low fat" and, without fortification, for "good source" of at least one of the following: dietary fiber, vitamin A, or vitamin C. This claim relates diets low in fat

Health Claim	Definition
	and rich in fruits and vegetables (and thus vitamins A and C and dietary fiber) to reduced cancer risk. FDA authorized this claim in place of an antioxidant vitamin and cancer claim.
Folic acid and neural tube defects	Foods must meet or exceed criteria for "good source" of folate: at least 40 mcg of folic acid per serving (at least 10% of the Daily Value).
Dietary sugar alcohol and dental caries	Foods must meet the criteria for "sugar free." The sugar alcohol must be xylitol, sorbitol, mannitol, maltitol, isomalt, lactitol, hydrogenated starch hydrolysates, hydrogenated glucose syrups, erythritol, or a combination of these.
Dietary soluble fiber, such as that found in whole oats and psyllium seed husk, and coronary heart disease	Foods must meet criteria for "low saturated fat," "low cholesterol," and "low fat." Foods that contain whole oats must contain at least 0.75 g of soluble fiber per serving. Foods that contain psyllium seed husk must contain at least 1.7 g of soluble fiber per serving.
Diets low in saturated fat and cholesterol that include 25 grams of soy protein a day may reduce the risk of heart disease	Foods that carry the claim must also meet the criteria for "low fat," "low saturated fat," and "low cholesterol" content except the foods made with the whole soybean may also qualify for the health claim if they contain no fat in addition to that present in the whole soybean.
Plant sterol or plant stanol esters may help to reduce the risk of CHD	Foods containing at least 0.65 grams per serving of plant sterol esters [used in some margarine-like spreads and salad dressings, i.e. Benecol and Take Control], eaten twice a day with meals for a daily total intake of at least 1.3 grams, as part of a diet low in saturated fat and cholesterol, may reduce the risk of heart disease.

Setting Goals

You've just read hundreds of tips on eating healthier. Don't feel that you have to make a lot of changes in one fell swoop. Set realistic goals for yourself.

To set goals, you'll first want to find out what your current eating habits are. The best way is to record what you eat. Keep this food diary for a few days. Include the weekend and a couple of weekdays. You may be asked to do this before your first visit with a dietitian.

Here's what you'll want to write down:

■ Day.

■ Time of meal or snack.

■ Type of food and drink. How food was prepared (broiled, fried, steamed).

■ Amount of food and drink.

■ Notes of interest, for example: at a friend's house, in a restaurant, low blood glucose.

■ Optional: Feelings or stress related to the food intake.

With well-kept food records, you can identify habits you want to change. For example, from your food diary you see that you eat breakfast on the run from a fast-food spot or work cafeteria Monday through Friday. Your usual choices are a sausage biscuit, a bagel with regular cream cheese, or a mega-muffin.

You decide you want to eat healthier breakfasts. You're ready to set a goal. A goal should be:

■ *realistic*

■ *easy to achieve*

■ *specific in frequency*

■ *short in time span*

Goal "For the next two months (*short time frame*), three days each week (*specific frequency*), I will choose one of these healthier breakfasts: an English muffin with jelly and a small banana, or bagel with a thin layer of cream cheese with an orange (*realistic and easy to achieve*)."

Observation From your food diary, you and your dietitian notice you consume next to no milk or yogurt over the course of a week.

Goal "For the next month (*short time frame*), three days each week (*specific frequency*), I will buy a carton of fat-free milk with my lunch or take a container of refrigerated non-fat fruited yogurt to eat as dessert (*realistic and easy to achieve*)."

Record your goals. Keep them handy: in your calendar, on your refrigerator, on the mirror in your bathroom, or on your night table. Review your goals every few days.

At the end of the time frame you set, answer these questions: "Did I meet my goals? If not, why not? Were they unrealistic? Was the time frame too long?"

If you need to, redesign the goals to make them easier to accomplish or write another goal that you can achieve more easily.

If you met your goals, pat yourself on the back, then set new ones while you continue to practice the old ones.

You won't always stick to your new goals. Forgive yourself and get back on track as soon as possible. Some behaviors easily become second nature and others are more difficult to cement.

A HEALTHY LIFESTYLE IS WITHIN YOUR REACH

Step-by-step, one goal, two goals—the new habits are beginning to feel like second nature. You change other habits, one at a time. Your confidence and commitment grow. Your blood glucose levels approach your target ranges. You've got more trimming to do in the waistline, but the scale is headed downward. You feel proud of yourself. It's time for a reward: a weekend get-away, new clothes, or a membership at the local YMCA.

You are on the road to a healthier lifestyle!

Index

A

A, vitamin, 11, 96, 125, 168–169, 174
Acesulfame potassium (ace-k), 265
Adequate Intake (AI) levels, 7
Alcohol, 273–275
  effect on blood glucose, 273–274
  exchanges for, 275
  nutrition profile for, 275
Alitame, 266
All-American Tuna or Salmon, 204
Allium vegetables, 102
Almond-Pesto White Beans with
    Vegetables, 56
Almonds, 244
Alpha-tocopherols, 11
Amaranth, 28
American Association of Diabetes
    Educators, 295
American Diabetes Association
  Recognized Diabetes Education
    Programs, 295
  recommendations of, 11, 13–14, 16,
    20, 93, 177, 263, 273
American Dietetic Association, recom-
    mendations of, 20
Anemia, pernicious, 10
Angel Hair with Feta and Capers, 50
Antioxidants, from vegetables, 93
Apple Sandwiches, 146
Apples, 144–145
  serving tips, 145
  varieties of, 144
Arugula and Watercress Salad, 116
Asian Bean Salad, 61
Asian Noodle Salad, 47
Asian Scallop Fettucine, 49
Asian Tuna or Salmon, 204
Asian vegetable topping, for potatoes,
    rice, and pasta, 77
Aspartame, 265
  not for people with PKU, 265
Avocado, 240–241
  buying and storing, 240

B

B1, vitamin, 8
B2, vitamin, 9
B3, vitamin, 9
B5, vitamin, 9
B6, vitamin, 9
B12, vitamin, 10, 168, 174
Bagels, 27
Barley, 28
Barley and Brown Rice, 30
Basic Polenta, 40–41
Basic Quinoa, 33
Basic Wild Rice, 36
Bean Salad, 60–61
Beans, peas, and lentils, 53–69
  benefits of, 53
  buying and storing, 53–54
  cooking, 54–55
  exchanges for, 85
Beans, peas, and lentils recipes, 24
  Almond-Pesto White Beans with
    Vegetables, 56
  Bean Salad, 60–61
  Black Bean Jicama Salad, 62
  Bow Tie Pasta with Sun-Dried
    Tomato Pesto and White Beans,
    57
  Colorful Lentil Salad, 58
  Couscous Bean Pilaf, 69
  Herbed Chickpeas and Potatoes, 68
  Pasta Fagioli, 59
  Red Bean Creole, 65
  Shrimp and Bean Skillet, 67
  Spanish Black Bean Soup, 63

Tex-Mex Beans, 66
White Bean Chili, 64
Beef recipes, 182
Chinese Stir-fried Beef with Ginger, 226
Marinated Steak Kabobs, 225
Spiced Lamb Stew, 227
Berries, 129–130
buying and storing, 129
Berry Vinegar, 100
Beta carotene, 11
Biotin, 10
Black Bean Jicama Salad, 62
Blackberries, 129
Blood glucose
alcohol and, 273–274
protein and, 4
Blood lipid levels
controlling, 262
goals for people with diabetes, 160
risks associated with, 159–160
Blood pressure, 177–179
related to sodium, 177–178, 308
Blueberries, 129
Blueberries with Almond Cream, 131
Blueberry Lemon Muffins, 132
Bow Tie Pasta with Sun-Dried Tomato
Pesto and White Beans, 57
Brazil nuts, 244
Breads
exchanges for, 83
"whole-wheat," 26
Broccoli, 107
Broccoli and Garlic, 109
Broccoli with Sesame Seeds and
Scallions, 108
Brussels sprouts, 107
Brussels Sprouts with Chestnuts, 110
Buckwheat, 28
Butter vs. margarine, 239
Butternut Squash and Pear Soup, 82

C

C, vitamin, 10, 97, 102, 126, 137
Cabbage, 107
Calcium, 12
milk fortified with, 167–168
sources of, 166–170
soy milk fortified with, 174
Calorie ranges
menus for 1200–1400 per day, 277,
279–283
menus for 1600–1800 per day, 277,
284–288
menus for 2000–2200 per day, 277,
289–293
and weight loss objectives, 294
Calories from fat
burning, 261
on food labels, 162–163
Cancer, 308
Canola oil, 236–237
Cantaloupe, 137
Caramelized Onions, 104
Carbohydrate counting
advanced, 18–19
basic, 18
resources on, 19
ways of counting, 18–19
Carbohydrate-to-insulin ratio, 18
Carbohydrates, 1–3
exchanges for, 17
fiber, 3
and insulin, 2–3
keeping constant, 15
quantities of, 2
sources of, 2
sugars vs. starches, 1
Carob Brownies, 268
Carotenoids, 11
Cashews, 244
Cauliflower, 107

Cauliflower with Cheddar Cheese
Sauce, 111
Cereals
exchanges for, 83–84
fiber from, 155, 168
Change to healthier habits, 311
CHD. *See* Coronary heart disease
Cheese, 189–190
stretching, 189
Cheese Dressing with Low-fat Sour
Cream, 101
Cheese Polenta, 40
Chestnuts, 244–245
Chicken, 214
Chicken, Spinach, and Shell Soup, 51
Chicken and turkey, 214–222
buying and storing, 214–215
Chicken and turkey recipes, 182
Chicken Salad in 64+ Ways,
220–221
Chicken with Tri-colored Peppers,
218
Grilled Chicken Breasts with Fruit
Salsa, 219
Oriental Turkey Salad, 222
Wild Rice Sun-dried Cherry Stuffed
Chicken, 216–217
Chicken Salad in 64+ Ways, 220–221
Chicken with Tri-colored Peppers, 218
Chinese Chicken with Cashews, 247
Chinese Ginger Salmon, 199
Chinese Stir-fried Beef with Ginger,
226
Chive Corn Pudding, 79
Cholesterol, 159–161
in eggs, 228
on food labels, 163, 298, 300
Chromium, 14
Cioppino, 207
Citrus fruits, 130
buying and storing, 130

Claims
health, 307–309
nutrition, 304–307
Cobalamin, 10
Coconuts, 245
Cold Cucumber Sauce for Fish,
Low-Fat, 213
Collagen, 10
Colorful Lentil Salad, 58
Confetti Rice and Beans, 39
Cooking oils, 236–237
Cool Melon Soup, 141
Copper, 14
Corn, 28, 78
cooking, 78
selecting, 78
Cornish hens, 214
Coronary heart disease (CHD), 308–309
Counting. *See* Carbohydrate counting
Couscous, 32
Couscous Bean Pilaf, 69
Crackers
exchanges for, 84
fiber from, 155
Cranberry Rice, 42
Creamy Mashed Potatoes, 75
Creamy Spinach Dip, 252
Crispy Fish Filets, 212
Cruciferous vegetables, 107
Crunchy Shrimp and Broccoli Stir-fry,
206
Curried Cauliflower Soup, 112
Curry Couscous, 32
Curry Dressing with Low-fat Sour
Cream, 101
Cyclamate, 266

D
D, vitamin, 11, 168–170, 174
Daily values (DV), 29
on food labels, 298, 301–302

Dark leafy greens, 94, 107
buying and storing, 107
DASH. *See* Dietary Approaches to
Stop Hypertension Study
Deep red vegetables, 94
Deep yellow vegetables, 94
Diabetes, blood lipid goals for people
with, 160
Diabetes food pyramid, 20–21, 92, 122
Dietary Approaches to Stop
Hypertension (DASH) Study,
178–179
Dietary Reference Intakes (DRIs), 7–8
AI levels, 7
EARs, 7
RDAs, 7
ULs, 7
Dietitians
consulting with, 22
finding, 295–296
paying for, 295–296
DNA, creation of, 9, 13
DRIs. *See* Dietary Reference Intakes
Duck, 214

E

E, vitamin, 11–12, 244
EARs. *See* Estimated Average
Requirements
Easy Dressings with Low-fat Sour
Cream, 101
Eggs, 228–229
buying and storing, 228
cholesterol in, 228
cooking with, 229
"Enriched" grain products, 26
Enrichment Act of 1942, 8
Estimated Average Requirements
(EARs), 7
Exchanges
for alcohol, 275

for beans, peas, and lentils, 85
for breads, 83
for carbohydrates, 17
for cereals, 83–84
for crackers, 84
for fats, 17, 257–258
for fruits, 151–152
for grains, 83–85
for meat and meat substitutes, 17,
176, 230–234
for pasta, 85
for snacks, 84
for starchy vegetables, 85–86
for sweets, 271–272
system of, 15–18
for vegetables, 118–119
Eyeballing measurements, 88

F

Fad diets, 191
Fall Spinach Salad, 114
Fat replacers, 238
Fat-soluble vitamins, 11–12
vitamin A, 11, 96, 125
vitamin D, 11
vitamin E, 11–12
vitamin K, 12
Fats, 5, 159–163, 235–258
calories from, 162–163
exchanges for, 17
in meats and meat substitutes, 183
omega-3, in seafood and fish, 198
replacing, 238
risks associated with, 159–160
varieties of, 160–162, 236–238
Fats recipes, 235
Chinese Chicken with Cashews,
247
Herbed Avocado Dressing, 241
New Waldorf Salad, 246
Whole-Wheat Flax Loaf, 243

FDA. *See* U.S. Food and Drug Administration
Festive Sweet Potatoes, 72
Fiber, 153–158, 308–309
   adding, 155–157
   adjusting insulin for, 158
   benefits of, 3
   sources of, 153–154
Figs, 128
Filberts, 245
Fish. *See also* Seafood and fish
   choosing lean, 188
Flavored Vinegars, 100
Flax oil and seeds, 242–243
Fluoride, 14
Foil-Roasted Herb Potatoes, 74
Folate/folic acid, 9–10, 309
   sources for, 96, 244
Food labels, 88, 157, 297–309
   contents of, 298–304
   different formats for, 303–304
   health claims on, 307–309
Food pyramid. *See* Diabetes food pyramid
Food scale, 88
Foods to limit, 179
"Fortified" grain products, 27
French Bean Salad, 61
French topping, for potatoes, rice, and pasta, 77
French Tuna or Salmon, 204
Fructose, 263
Fruit juice, 124–125
Fruit Shakes, 172
Fruits, 121–163
   benefits of, 123–124
   berries, 129–130
   cautions regarding, 127
   citrus, 130
   exchanges for, 151–152
   fanciful, 128, 137
   fresh, frozen, canned, or dried, 126
   as sources of fiber, 154
Fruits recipes, 121
   Apple Sandwiches, 146
   Blueberries with Almond Cream, 131
   Blueberry Lemon Muffins, 132
   Cool Melon Soup, 141
   Grapefruit Combo Salad, 136
   Island Sundaes, 150
   Lime Guacamole with Mango, 138
   Mango Chicken Salad, 140
   Minted Kiwi Salad, 143
   Orange and Fennel Salad, 135
   Orange and Kiwi Salad, 142
   Pan-Seared Pork with Mango Salsa, 139
   Pears Baked with White Wine, 149
   Red Cherry Frozen Yogurt Sundae, 147
   Red Grape and Turkey Salad, 148
   Strawberry-Peach Soup, 133
   Strawberry Raspberry Almond Shake, 134
Fruity Yogurt Cheese, 173
Fusilli with Sage and Peppers, 44

G

Glazed Parsnips, 81
Glycemic Index, 21
Goal setting, 311–312
Grain products, 23, 25–42
   bagels, 27
   breads from, 26–27
   cooking, 29
   "enriched," 26
   exchanges for, 83–85
   "fortified," 27
   varieties of, 28
   wheat germ, 29
   whole, 28–29

Grains recipes, 23
    Barley and Brown Rice, 30
    Basic Polenta, 40–41
    Basic Quinoa, 33
    Basic Wild Rice, 36
    Confetti Rice and Beans, 39
    Couscous, 32
    Cranberry Rice, 42
    Italian Wild Rice Pilaf, 38
    Nutty Blueberry Pancakes, 31
    Quinoa Salad, 35
    Quinoa Stuffed Peppers, 34
    Wild Rice Salad, 37
Grapefruit Combo Salad, 136
Greek topping, for potatoes, rice, and
    pasta, 77
Green Beans with Tomatoes and
    Herbs, 105
Greens, dark leafy, 94, 107
Grilled Chicken Breasts with Fruit
    Salsa, 219
Grilled Polenta, 41

H

HDL ("good") cholesterol, 159–160
Health claims, on food labels, 307–309
Health insurance, paying for a dietitian,
    295–296
Healthy Coleslaw, 113
Healthy lifestyle, 311–312
Heart disease, risks of, 159–160
Herb Barley and Brown Rice, 30
Herb Dressing with Low-fat Sour
    Cream, 101
Herb Polenta, 40
Herb Vinegar, 100
Herb Yogurt Cheese, 173
Herbed Avocado Dressing, 241
Herbed Chickpeas and Potatoes, 68
Honey, 263
Hot Artichoke Dip, 250

Hummus, 251
Hydrogenated fats, 237–238
Hypoglycemia, 273–274

I

Indian Bean Salad, 61
Insoluble fiber, 153
Insulin. *See also* Carbohydrate-to-
    insulin ratio
    adjusting for fiber, 158
    carbohydrates and, 2–3
Iodine, 13
Iron, 12–13
Island Sundaes, 150
Isoflavones, 192
Italian Bean Salad, 61
Italian Couscous, 32
Italian Tuna or Salmon, 204
Italian Wild Rice Pilaf, 38
Italiano topping, for potatoes, rice, and
    pasta, 77

J

Just Peachy Crisp, 270

K

K, vitamin, 12
Kiwi, 137

L

Labels. *See* Food labels
Lactose intolerance, handling, 170
LDL ("bad") cholesterol, 159–161
Leafy greens, dark, 94, 107
Lean cuts, choosing, 188, 223
Lemon Raisin Barley and Brown
    Rice, 30
Lentils. *See* Beans, peas, and lentils
Lime Guacamole with Mango, 138
Low- to no-calorie sweeteners,
    265–267
    blends of, 266

Low-fat Buffalo Wings, 256
Low-Fat Sauces for Fish, 213
Lower-fat party foods recipes, 235
    Creamy Spinach Dip, 252
    Hot Artichoke Dip, 250
    Hummus, 251
    Low-fat Buffalo Wings, 256
    Open-faced Mini Bagel Bar, 254–255
    Potato Skin Bar, 253
    Smoky Cheese Dip, 249
    Sun-dried Tomato Spread, 248
    Tomato Pizza Bagels, 255
    Turkey Chutney Sandwiches, 255
    Veggie Sandwich, 254
Lycopene, 102

M

Macadamia nuts, 245
Magnesium, 13, 168, 244
Mango Chicken Salad, 140
Mangoes, 137
    buying and storing, 137
Marbling, in meats, 223
Margarine, 239
Marinara Sauce, 52
Marinated Steak Kabobs, 225
Meal planning approaches, 15–22
    carbohydrate counting, 18–19
    diabetes food pyramid, 20–21
    exchange lists for, 16–18
    Glycemic Index, 21
    myths about, 15–16
    selecting among, 22
    snacks in, 278
Measuring
    cups and spoons for, 87–88
    hand guides for, 89
Meat and meat substitutes, 181–234,
    223–227
    buying, 224
    choosing lean, 188

    cutting back on, 187–188
    exchanges for, 17
    fats in, 183
    grades of, 223
    protein in, 183–187
    raw *vs.* cooked, 224
Meat and meat substitutes recipes,
    181–182
"Medical nutrition therapy," 295
Medicare, 295–296
Menu planning, 277–296
    carbohydrates in, 277–278
    fats in, 278
    for healthy eating, 279–294
    meat in, 278
    milk in, 278
    snacks in, 278
Mexicali topping, for potatoes, rice,
    and pasta, 77
Mexican Bean Salad, 61
Middle Eastern Tuna Salad, 203
Milk, 165–179
    fortified with calcium, 167–168
Milk and yogurt recipes, 165
    Fruit Shakes, 172
    Shrimp and Corn Bisque, 171
    Soy Milk Smoothie, 175
    Yogurt Cheese, 173
Millet, 28
Minerals, 12–14
    calcium, 12
    chromium, 14
    copper, 14
    fluoride, 14
    on food labels, 298, 302
    iodine, 13
    iron, 12–13
    magnesium, 13
    phosphorus, 13
    selenium, 14
    zinc, 13–14

Minted Kiwi Salad, 143
Monounsaturated fats, 160, 236–237
　　exchanges for, 257
　　on food labels, 163
Muscle building, 191

N

NAS. *See* National Academy of
　　Sciences
Nateglinide, 19
National Academy of Sciences (NAS),
　　Food and Nutrition Board of, 7–8,
　　11
Neotame, 266
New Orleans Shrimp Creole, 210
New Waldorf Salad, 246
Niacin, 9
Non-nutritive sweeteners. *See* Low- to
　　no-calorie sweeteners
NutraSweet, 265
Nutrients, 1–5
　　carbohydrates, 1–3
　　fat, 5
　　from fruit, 126
　　protein, 3–5
Nutrition claims, 304–307
Nutrition Facts label, 88, 157, 298–299
　　contents of, 162–163, 298–204
Nuts, 244–247
　　buying and storing, 244
Nutty Barley and Brown Rice, 30
Nutty Blueberry Pancakes, 31
Nutty Yogurt Cheese, 173

O

Old-fashioned Spiced Banana Bread,
　　269
Olive oil, 236–237
Omega-3 fats, 160
　　in flax, 242
　　in seafood and fish, 194, 198

Open-faced Mini Bagel Bar, 254–255
Orange and Fennel Salad, 135
Orange and Kiwi Salad, 142
Orange Dressing with Low-fat Sour
　　Cream, 101
Oriental Turkey Salad, 222
Oven-dried Tomatoes, Garlic, and
　　Pasta, 48

P

Pan-Seared Pork with Mango Salsa,
　　139
Pantothenic acid, 9
Papayas, 128
Party foods. *See* Lower-fat party foods
　　recipes
Pasta, 43–52
　　cooking, 43
　　exchanges for, 85
　　new ways with, 43
　　toppings for, 77
Pasta Fagioli, 59
Pasta Primavera, 45
Pasta recipes, 23
　　Angel Hair with Feta and Capers, 50
　　Asian Noodle Salad, 47
　　Asian Scallop Fettucine, 49
　　Chicken, Spinach, and Shell Soup, 51
　　Fusilli with Sage and Peppers, 44
　　Marinara Sauce, 52
　　Oven-dried Tomatoes, Garlic, and
　　　Pasta, 48
　　Pasta Primavera, 45
　　Penne Pasta with Basil Vinaigrette, 46
　　Pesto Sauce, 52
Peanuts, 245
Pears Baked with White Wine, 149
Peas, 54. *See also* Beans, peas, and
　　lentils
Pecans, 245
Penne Pasta with Basil Vinaigrette, 46

Percentage daily values, on food labels, 298, 301
Pernicious anemia, 10
Pesto Sauce, 52
Phenylketonuria (PKU), aspartame not for people with, 265
Phosphorus, 13, 168
Phytochemicals, 93–94
Pine nuts, 245
Pineapples, 128
Pistachios, 245
PKU. *See* Phenylketonuria
Polyols, 263–265
Polyunsaturated fats, 160, 237
    exchanges for, 257–258
    on food labels, 163
Pomegranates, 128
Portion control, 87–89
    tips for, 88–89, 123–124, 190
    tools for, 87–88
Potassium, 168, 244
Potato Skin Bar, 253
Potatoes, 73. *See also* Sweet potatoes
    cooking, 73
    selecting, 73
    toppings for, 77
    varieties of, 73
Poultry, 214–222
    choosing lean, 188
    cooking, 215
Prandin, 19
Pregnancy
    importance of folic acid in, 9–10
    saccharin in, 265
Protein, 3–5
    and blood glucose, 4
    controlling portions with, 190
    lightening up on, 184–187
    in meats and meat substitutes, 183–187
    quantities of, 4
    sources of, 5
    stretching, 187
Pyridoxine, 9

Q

Quinoa, 28
Quinoa Salad, 35
Quinoa Stuffed Peppers, 34

R

Raspberries, 129
RDAs. *See* Recommended Dietary Allowances
RDIs. *See* Reference Daily Intakes
Recipes
    for beans, peas, and lentils, 24
    for beef, 182
    for chicken and turkey, 182
    for fats, 235
    for fruits, 121
    for grains, 23
    for lower-fat party foods, 235
    for meat and meat substitutes, 181–182
    for milk and yogurt, 165
    for pasta, 23
    for seafood and fish, 181
    for soy, 181
    for starchy vegetables, 24
    for sugars, sweets, and sweeteners, 259
    for vegetables, 91
Recommended Dietary Allowances (RDAs), 7, 29
    for protein, 4, 184
Record-keeping, 312
Red Bean Creole, 65
Red Cherry Frozen Yogurt Sundae, 147
Red Grape and Turkey Salad, 148
Reference Daily Intakes (RDIs), 8, 102, 302

Repaglinide, 19
Riboflavin, 9, 168
Rice, 28
    toppings for, 77
RNA, creation of, 9, 13
Roasted Garlic, 103
Roasted Soy Nuts, 195
Rye, 28

S

Saccharin, 265–266
    not using in pregnancy, 265
Salads, 97–99
    dressing, 99–101
    tips for, 97–98
Salmon, 198
Salsa Dressing with Low-fat Sour
    Cream, 101
Salt, blood pressure related to, 178
Saturated fats, 160, 237–238
    exchanges for, 258
    on food labels, 163, 298, 300
Seafood and fish, 197–213
    buying and storing, 197–198
    omega-3 fats in, 198
Seafood and fish recipes, 181
    Chinese Ginger Salmon, 199
    Cioppino, 207
    Crispy Fish Filets, 212
    Crunchy Shrimp and Broccoli Stir-
        fry, 206
    Low-Fat Sauces for Fish, 213
    Middle Eastern Tuna Salad, 203
    New Orleans Shrimp Creole, 210
    Seafood Kabobs Hawaiian, 208
    Seared Salmon with Asparagus and
        Green Onion, 200
    Seared Sesame Tuna with Orange
        Glaze, 201
    Shrimp Scampi, 211
    Stir-Fry Fish, 209

    Teriyaki Glazed Tuna, 202
    Ways With Tuna or Salmon, 204–205
Seafood Kabobs Hawaiian, 208
Seared Salmon with Asparagus and
    Green Onion, 200
Seared Sesame Tuna with Orange
    Glaze, 201
Selenium, 14
Serving size. *See also* Portion control
    on food labels, 298–300
Shrimp and Bean Skillet, 67
Shrimp and Corn Bisque, 171
Shrimp Scampi, 211
Smoky Cheese Dip, 249
Snacks, exchanges for, 84
Sodium
    blood pressure related to, 177–178
    on food labels, 298, 301
Soluble fiber, 153
Soy food, 192–196
    tempeh, 194
    tofu, 193–194
Soy Kale, 115
Soy milk, 169, 174
    fortified, 174
Soy Milk Smoothie, 175
Soy recipes, 181
    Roasted Soy Nuts, 195
    Teriyaki Tofu Kebobs, 196
Spanish Black Bean Soup, 63
Spenda, 266
Spiced Lamb Stew, 227
Spicy Vinegar, 100
Spinach Sauté with Mushrooms, 117
Starches, 23–89
    benefits of, 25
    vs. sugars, 1
Starchy vegetables, 70–82
    corn, 78
    exchanges for, 85–86
    potatoes, 73, 77

as sources of fiber, 153
sweet potatoes, 70
Starchy vegetables recipes, 24
   Butternut Squash and Pear Soup, 82
   Chive Corn Pudding, 79
   Creamy Mashed Potatoes, 75
   Festive Sweet Potatoes, 72
   Foil-Roasted Herb Potatoes, 74
   Glazed Parsnips, 81
   Sweet Potato Fries, 71
   Twice-Baked Potatoes, 76
   Vegetable Burritos, 80
Starlix, 19
Stir-Fry Fish, 209
Strawberries, 129
Strawberry-Peach Soup, 133
Strawberry Raspberry Almond Shake, 134
Sucralose, 266
Sugar alcohols, 263–265, 309
Sugar-free sweeteners, 263
Sugars
   on food labels, 298, 301
   vs. starches, 1
Sugars, sweets, and sweeteners, 259–275
   ADA recommendations, 260–262
   definitions, 260, 263
   tips for limiting, 262
Sugars, sweets, and sweeteners recipes, 259
   Carob Brownies, 268
   Just Peachy Crisp, 270
   Old-fashioned Spiced Banana Bread, 269
Sun-dried Tomato Spread, 248
Sweet Couscous, 32
Sweet Potato Fries, 71
Sweet potatoes, 70
   buying and storing, 70
Sweet tooth, satisfying, 262
Sweet Yogurt Cheese, 173

Sweets and sweeteners, 259–275
   low- to no-calorie, 265–267

T

Tartar Sauce for Fish, Low-Fat, 213
Tempeh, 194
Teriyaki Glazed Tuna, 202
Teriyaki Tofu Kebobs, 196
Tex Mex Barley and Brown Rice, 30
Tex-Mex Beans, 66
Thiamin, 8
Thirst quenchers, 120, 124–125
Thyroid hormones, 13
Tocopherols, 11
Tofu, 184, 193–194
Tolerable Upper Intake Levels (ULs), 7
Tomato Pizza Bagels, 255
Tomatoes, 102
   buying and storing, 102
Toppings, for potatoes, rice, and pasta, 77
Total carbohydrate
   on food labels, 298, 300
   polyols as part of, 264
Total cholesterol, 159–160
Total fat grams, on food labels, 163, 298, 300
Trans fats, 237–238
Triglycerides, 159–160
Tuna, 198
Turkey, 214
Turkey Chutney Sandwiches, 255
Twice-Baked Potatoes, 76

U

ULs. *See* Tolerable Upper Intake Levels
Ultraviolet light, 9
Upper Intake Levels (ULs), tolerable, 7
U.S. Department of Agriculture (USDA), 20, 168, 297
U.S. Food and Drug Administration (FDA), 124, 192, 265, 297, 307
U.S. Public Health Service, 16

V

Vegetable Burritos, 80
Vegetable Couscous, 32
Vegetables, 91–120
  allium, 102
  antioxidants from, 93
  benefits of, 93
  cooking, 95
  cruciferous, 107
  dark leafy greens, 107
  exchanges for, 118–119
  fresh, frozen, or canned, 95–96
  shopping for, 94–95
  as sources of fiber, 154
  starchy, 70–82
  tomatoes, 102
  vitamins from, 96–97
Vegetables recipes, 91
  Arugula and Watercress Salad, 116
  Broccoli and Garlic, 109
  Broccoli with Sesame Seeds and
    Scallions, 108
  Brussels Sprouts with Chestnuts, 110
  Caramelized Onions, 104
  Cauliflower with Cheddar Cheese
    Sauce, 111
  Curried Cauliflower Soup, 112
  Easy Dressings with Low-fat Sour
    Cream, 101
  Fall Spinach Salad, 114
  Flavored Vinegars, 100
  Green Beans with Tomatoes and
    Herbs, 105
  Healthy Coleslaw, 113
  Roasted Garlic, 103
  Soy Kale, 115
  Spinach Sauté with Mushrooms, 117
  Zucchini Marinara, 106
Veggie Sandwich, 254
Vitamins, 7–14
  fat-soluble, 11–12

  on food labels, 298, 302
  sources of, 8, 96–97, 125–126
  water-soluble, 8–10

W

Walnuts, 245
Water, 120
Water-soluble vitamins, 8–10
  biotin, 10
  folate/folic acid, 9–10
  vitamin B1, thiamin, 8
  vitamin B2, riboflavin, 9
  vitamin B3, niacin, 9
  vitamin B5, pantothenic acid, 9
  vitamin B6, pyridoxine, 9
  vitamin B12, cobalamin, 10
  vitamin C, 10, 97, 126
Ways With Tuna or Salmon, 204–205
Weight reduction, 177
  and alcohol, 274
  and calorie ranges, 294
Wheat, 28
Wheat germ, 29
  buying and storing, 29
White Bean Chili, 64
White Beans with Vegetables, 56
Whole grains, 28–29
"Whole-wheat" bread, 26
Whole-Wheat Flax Loaf, 243
Wild rice, 28
Wild Rice Salad, 37
Wild Rice Sun-dried Cherry Stuffed
    Chicken, 216–217

Y

Yogurt, 165–179
Yogurt Cheese, 173

Z

Zinc, 13–14
Zucchini Marinara, 106

About the American Diabetes Association

The American Diabetes Association is the nation's leading voluntary health organization supporting diabetes research, information, and advocacy. Its mission is to prevent and cure diabetes and to improve the lives of all people affected by diabetes. The American Diabetes Association is the leading publisher of comprehensive diabetes information. Its huge library of practical and authoritative books for people with diabetes covers every aspect of self-care, cooking and nutrition, fitness, weight control, medications, complications, emotional issues, and general self-care.

To order American Diabetes Association books: Call 1-800-232-6733. http://store.diabetes.org [Note: there is no need to use **www** when typing this particular Web address]

To join the American Diabetes Association: Call 1-800-806-7801. www.diabetes.org/membership

For more information about diabetes or ADA programs and services: Call 1-800-342-2383. E-mail: Customerservice@diabetes.org www.diabetes.org

To locate an ADA/NCQA Recognized Provider of quality diabetes care in your area: Call 1-703-549-1500 ext. 2202. www.diabetes.org/recognition/Physicians/ListAll.asp

To find an ADA Recognized Education Program in your area: Call 1-888-232-0822. www.diabetes.org/recognition/education.asp

To join the fight to increase funding for diabetes research, end discrimination, and improve insurance coverage: Call 1-800-342-2383. www.diabetes.org/advocacy

To find out how you can get involved with the programs in your community: Call 1-800-342-2383. See below for program Web addresses.

- *American Diabetes Month:* Educational activities aimed at those diagnosed with diabetes—month of November. www.diabetes.org/ADM

- *American Diabetes Alert:* Annual public awareness campaign to find the undiagnosed—held the fourth Tuesday in March. www.diabetes.org/alert

- *The Diabetes Assistance & Resources Program (DAR):* diabetes awareness program targeted to the Latino community. www.diabetes.org/DAR

- *African American Program:* diabetes awareness program targeted to the African American community. www.diabetes.org/africanamerican

- *Awakening the Spirit: Pathways to Diabetes Prevention & Control:* diabetes awareness program targeted to the Native American community. www.diabetes.org/awakening

To find out about an important research project regarding type 2 diabetes: www.diabetes.org/ada/research.asp

To obtain information on making a planned gift or charitable bequest: Call 1-888-700-7029. www.diabetes.org/ada/plan.asp

To make a donation or memorial contribution: Call 1-800-342-2383. www.diabetes.org/ada/cont.asp